Change How You See,
Not How You Look

Change How You See, Not How You Look

Power Tools For Celebrating Your Body

J. Alison Hilber

Trafford Publishing
A Division of Trafford Holdings Ltd.
Victoria, BC, Canada

Cover design by Cybèle Elaine Werts

Book design by Nicholas Vittum.

National Library of Canada Cataloguing in Publication

Hilber, J. Alison (Jan Alison), 1951-
  Change how you see, not how you look : power tools for celebrating your body /
  J. Alison Hilber.
  ISBN 1-55369-341-8
  1. Body image in women. 2. Overweight women--Psychology.
3. Obesity in women--Psychological aspects.
4. Self-esteem in women. I. Title.
BF697.5.B63H54 2002   158.1'082   C2002-901426-3

TRAFFORD

This book was published *on-demand* in cooperation with Trafford Publishing.
On-demand publishing is a unique process and service of making a book available for retail sale to the public taking advantage of on-demand manufacturing and Internet marketing.
On-demand publishing includes promotions, retail sales, manufacturing, order fulfilment, accounting and collecting royalties on behalf of the author.

Suite 6E, 2333 Government St., Victoria, B.C. V8T 4P4, CANADA

Phone	250-383-6864	Toll-free	1-888-232-4444 (Canada & US)
Fax	250-383-6804	E-mail	sales@trafford.com
Web site	www.trafford.com	TRAFFORD PUBLISHING IS A DIVISION OF TRAFFORD HOLDINGS LTD.	
Trafford Catalogue #02-0154		www.trafford.com/robots/02-0154.html	

10   9   8   7   6   5   4   3   2   1

To my mother, Beverly,
my sister, Marcia
my niece, Sara
and all women everywhere,
no matter where you are on your journey

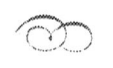

Contents

Power Tool Box .... *ix*
Acknowledgments .... *xii*
Introduction .... *xiv*

From Goddess to Victim 1
Cultural Awareness—Where We Live 5
Personal Awareness—Who We Are 9
Mind Awareness—What We Think 13
Body Awareness—How We Feel 21
Spiritual Awareness—How We Love 29
Relationships 37
Health 43
Role Modeling 53
Healing Ourselves 59
Healing the Culture 71
From Victim to Goddess 75

Appendix: Alison's Musings *79*

Why Celebrate Your Body? *80*
"You Can't Be a Beacon" *82*
Will Power v. Self-care *85*
Free to Be: Thin v. Happy *88*
Gratitude and Forgiveness *92*
Emotional Poker *96*
Passion Is an Inside Job *100*
Walk When You Want To Walk *103*
Being Extraordinary *106*
Walking the Path *109*
Four Agreements with Your Body *113*

References *117*
About the author *121*

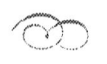

Power Tool Box

CHAPTER 1: FROM GODDESS TO VICTIM
  Power Tool: *I am already beautiful* 3

CHAPTER 2: CULTURAL AWARENESS
  Power Tools:
    1. *Awareness* 6
    2. *Acceptance* 7
    3. *Action* 7

CHAPTER 3: PERSONAL AWARENESS
  Power Tools:
    1. *Quiet your mind* 10
    2. *Write your own "herstory"* 11
    3. *Know your body* 11

CHAPTER 4: MIND AWARENESS
  Power Tools:
    1. *If you wouldn't say it to someone else, then*
       you aren't allowed to say it to yourself 14
    2. *Throw away the scale* 15
    3. *Define yourself* 16
    4. *Identify your anger* 16
    5. *Live "as if"* 16
    6. *It's not about you* 18
    7. *Take responsibility* 19
    8. *Create affirmations* 20

CHAPTER 5: BODY AWARENESS
  Power Tools:
    1. *How are you caring for your body?* 22
    2. *Dialogue with your body* 27
    3. *Bodybuilding* 27

CHAPTER 6: SPIRITUAL AWARENESS

Power Tools:

1. Live in the moment 30
2. Create an altar 31
3. Breathe 31
4. No expectations and an open heart 32
5. Meditate—Relaxing Breath 32
6. Draw 35
7. Journal 35
8. Other tools 36

CHAPTER 7: RELATIONSHIPS

Power Tools:

1. First you, then them 38
2. Define what you want 38
3. Show up 39
4. Be naked often 39
5. Sex is not the enemy 40
6. Women united 42
7. Pamper your divine self 42

CHAPTER 8: HEALTH

Power Tools:

1. Envision health 46
2. Care of your body 46
    a. Movement 46
    b. Food 47
    c. Diets 48
    d. Care giver 48
3. Care of your mind 48
    a. The law of attraction 49
    b. Don't take it personally 49
4. Care of your spirit 50

CHAPTER 9: ROLE MODELING

Power Tools:

1. Seek out true role models 54

2. *Read affirming, joyful books* 54
3. *Throw away "beauty" magazines* 55
4. *Treat your children well* 55
5. *Communicate with your daughters* 56
6. *Communicate with your sons* 57
7. *Start young* 57
8. *Speak up, speak out* 58

CHAPTER 10: HEALING OURSELVES
Power Tools:
1. *Healing the mind* 60
   a. *Self-visualization* 60
   b. *Self-affirmation* 61
   c. *Create your own reality* 62
2. *Healing the heart* 63
   a. *Be grateful* 63
   b. *Be forgiving* 64
3. *Healing the spirit* 65
   a. *Stay present* 65
   b. *Release* 66
   c. *Play* 67
4. *Search for Wholeness* 67
   Wholeness Visualization 68

CHAPTER 11: HEALING THE CULTURE
Power Tools:
1. *Don't ignore men* 72
2. *Educate and encourage* 72
3. *Walk the walk* 73

CHAPTER 12: FROM VICTIM TO GODDESS
Power Tool: 77

We are the power in everyone;
We are the dance of the moon and the sun;
We are the hopes that will not hide;
We are the turning of the tide.

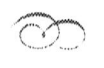

Acknowledgments

I look forward to the day when my work in this field is unnecessary. In the meantime, I wish to express my deepest gratitude to all of the teachers in my life who have helped me grow in love and compassion and forgiveness, allowing me to be bold and visible and self-loving.

My gratitude and love to:

Meghan O'Brien McDermott. . . dear friend, fellow traveler, inspiration, and first reader. You have her to thank for the loss of 23 boring and egotistical pages of original manuscript. Be grateful, be very grateful. I know I am.

Cybèle Elaine Werts, for her imagination and creativity in designing my website and my book cover, and for her constant presence and support in my life.

Nicholas Vittum. . . dear friend and one of the men who "gets it." Also, my layout artist, completely responsible for the form and structure of the words within.

McNeil, Leddy & Sheahan, for providing me with a steady, fun, accepting and supportive day-job environment, which was essential to my staying warm, dry and well-fed while pursuing this project.

Burlington College, for providing me with a solid alternative education and wise and caring guidance that allowed me to explore my true calling and begin the manifestation of my dreams long before graduation.

Trafford Publishing, for making the publication and distribution of that dream possible.

My very best friend, Marie-Andrée Gervais and all my other dear friends and family who have encouraged, supported and unconditionally loved me through every leg of my journey thus far.

Finally, I honor and bless all the women in this country who have endured the harassment of rigid, patriarchal beauty standards and are now ready to stand tall, take responsibility for their own happiness, and celebrate their bodies and themselves for the Goddesses they are.

Alison
February 2002

Introduction

CELEBRATE: *(sel´-e-brat) v.* To observe with ceremonies
of respect, festivity and rejoicing; to extol or praise.
— *The American Heritage Dictionary, 3ᵈ edition,* 1994

CELEBRATION: That's the goal. To find ourselves respecting, rejoicing and praising our bodies in all their glory, no
matter what size, shape, age or ability we are blessed to be. This
requires lightness and depth, inside and outside joy, a longing to
know and accept ourselves just as we are, and a belief that all we
have to do is remember that we are worthy of love and capable
of giving it unconditionally to ourselves. This book is offered as
a guide for that journey.

This process is not about figuring out *why* we look the way
we do. There are no strategies here for dieting or for how to
manage our emotions so we don't eat or insinuations that being
fat is about not loving ourselves. Emotional issues can sometimes lead to excess fat (meaning above your natural weight)
and many of us use food as a drug. But being shamed and feeling guilty only compounds those issues. In most cases, being fat
is just another way to be. This process is about changing the way
we see, not the way we look. Once our self-view changes, the

issues regarding our emotional relationship with food will naturally adjust to their healthiest place, because self-care will no
longer require will power. Self-care only requires self-love.

Scientists say that if 11% of a society's members change their
mind, there will be a cultural shift. Eleven percent is very attain-
able. But it must begin inside each one of us, something I will
be repeating throughout the book. *Your* mind must change;
your energy in the world must shift; *your* inner light must shine.
Then, and only then, can you hope to have any influence on the
larger reality. But, first things first.

This is a book about choices and the tools to help you make
the ones best suited to you. There is no reason that you can't
love yourself no matter what you look like and make choices
only as they suit your *own* higher purpose. It is from this center
of self-loving energy that you will manifest your true self in the
Universe. The only way to change anything is to begin inside
yourself. You do have control, but only of your own process,
thoughts, actions, and beliefs. The first thing to know is that
CHOICE is the most powerful tool of all. How you choose to
see, how you choose to react, who and what you choose to believe, how and who you choose to BE—every part of your life
experience is about choices.

Finally, it is important to understand that this book is not
about big bodies being better than small bodies. It is about small
bodies *not* being better than big bodies. It is about *no* bodies
being better than *any other* bodies. And though the emphasis
may seem to be on size, please be assured that no matter what
issues you have about your appearance, whether it be weight,
age, facial hair, baldness or bowed legs, this book can help you
see through different eyes and find your true inner vision.

Change How You See, Not How You Look provides Power
Tools at the end of every chapter . . . little hints, affirmations,
rituals, ways of helping you deal with the culture, the media,
belief systems, relationships, spirituality, the body/mind/spirit
split, and healing. There are tools to deconstruct what you

believe about women in general and yourself in particular, and tools to help you rebuild, remember, and restore the integrity and inherent beauty of your body and your spirit so you can begin joyfully celebrating every part of your being.

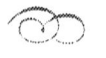

From Goddess to Victim

*The most important beauty secret is to remember you are
already beautiful.*

—Bobbi Brown, Makeup Artist

The dictionary describes FAT in many ways. Indeed, one set
of definitions is "obesity, corpulence; unnecessary excess." What
you might not know is that the majority of the definitions are
along these lines: "the best or richest part; abounding in desirable elements; fertile or productive; rich; lucrative; prosperous;
wealthy." Clearly, the word fat needs a new public relations
agent. How have we managed to twist the "best or richest" into
something so terrifying that some of us are willing to die rather
than be it?

It is a rare woman who doesn't or hasn't disliked her body,
no matter what size she is. And how could she not. Daily, we are
blasted with messages from all directions—magazines, television, billboards, movies, neighbors, friends, family—that we
can't be happy if we don't change x y z about our body or appearance. Body image becomes an increasingly fragile element
in our lives that begins taking up an enormous amount of our
energy, not to mention our dollars.

So, what exactly is "body image"? Is it just our physical size,
weight, ability? Does it encompass also the ways in which we

move in the world, our posture, how our bodies are adorned, what we feel comfortable doing, where we are comfortable being? It is all this, and more. It can be about our hair color, our height, our ethnicity, our sexual orientation, our age, our physical ability, our skin color, the tilt of our nose, the width of our mouth, the straightness of our teeth . . . as well, of course, as the size, shape and texture of our hips, thighs, breasts, hands, waist, toes, butts, ears, necks or heads!

As with all of life, body image is about perception: how we perceive ourselves, how society perceives us, how others perceive us, and how we perceive others perceiving us. For women, physical appearance and self-esteem are almost inextricably connected, and most of us in this culture struggle with various body image issues, even those who actually represent society's feminine "ideal." We are not thin enough, not pretty enough, not fit enough . . . not good enough. By internalizing these messages, we have learned to ignore our own beauty, our own worth, our own uniqueness in the Universe. Our self-esteem becomes intimately entwined with our self-image and, in this society, that image is almost always found lacking and in need of improvement. Our souls are depleted and our lives become limited.

One thing we can always count on is that, no matter what other appearance issues we may have, the perception of being fat will always carry the biggest stigma. It invokes the most dreaded fears. Most women would rather die than be fat . . . and many do. Incidences of eating disorders in the U.S. are skyrocketing and girls as young as nine years old are already dieting.

Continuing to be a victim of the cultural paradigm of thinness-above-all-else requires your cooperation. Moving out of victimhood requires taking responsibility for yourself. This process is about becoming aware and conscious of your choices and deciding for yourself who you want to be in the world. The bottom line is unconditional, unadulterated self-love. Hating your body desecrates the temple you live in and is the antithesis of self-love, which is the most essential element to health, joy

and spiritual growth. Once you begin that journey, you won't
believe the incredibly wonderful ways you will define yourself.
Your job, then, is to forget the external forces for a while and go
inside yourself. You must begin gathering the pieces of your
scattered self and bring them back together, allowing them to
work together to remind you of your own perfection in every
moment.

POWER TOOL:

REPEAT AS OFTEN AS POSSIBLE:

I Am Already Beautiful!

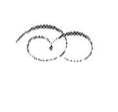

Cultural Awareness— Where We Live

The biggest fat lie of all . . . is that we have a weight problem. The truth is this:
WE don't have a weight problem: SOCIETY does.
—Cheri Erdman, *Nothing to Lose*, 1995

Awareness is vital to the beginning of any process of change. Awareness of who you are, where you come from, where you want to go, and what keeps you from moving forward. So, it is important to be aware of the messages that are being constantly put into the airwaves for you to take in. Only by being aware of how these messages sound, look and feel can you begin to consciously tune out the ones that make you feel bad about yourself.

The most obvious of these messages come from the media. This includes television, billboards, radio ads, newspaper ads, magazines, movies, store window displays. All these messages are designed to make us dissatisfied with ourselves so we will spend our money on one or more of the millions of items out there designed to make us look better, which we think will make us feel better. It is all about marketing. It is completely within the best interests of the American economy to keep women believing that we will never be thin enough, pretty enough, loved enough, happy enough, or good enough without whatever product we are being sold. These messages keep us hoping that just one more product, one more diet, one more gym membership, one more cosmetic will be the one that makes everything better. They sell us the false idea that happiness is right around their corner, and we spend billions of dollars, hours of time and undetermined energy a year hoping this will be true.

There are also the more subtle, indirect messages we receive about not fitting in. Mostly they come in the form of "average" things that are just too small for us: like seats in a theater or on a plane, many public bathroom stalls, and the gowns they give you at the doctor's office—all places that have the potential for real public embarrassment. Finally, there are all those mixed messages that appear everywhere: diets and dessert recipes on the same page of the magazine; a diet system ad next to an article about the increase in anorexia; headlines about finding our self-esteem placed next to a picture of a rail-thin model in a bikini touting the latest exercise craze; women in their underwear selling eyeliner. They are endless.

POWER TOOLS:

1. *Awareness:* The more aware you are that all of these messages exist, the easier it will be to replace them with your own mantras of self-love and joy. The more aware you are, the sooner you can face the dilemma, change the old tapes in your head and find your own voice again. Pay attention to the ads you see and notice the ways in which they may be directly or subliminally undermining your self-esteem, making you feel not good enough, not thin enough, not beautiful enough, not smart enough. By being aware of how the media tries to control and manipulate you, you can stop buying into it—literally and figuratively. Notice, as well, the few brilliant ads that encourage diversity and individuality and a strong sense of self, and support those markets.

2. *Acceptance:* Awareness also requires you to face your fears and anger at being so willing to cooperate with your own imprisonment. It is good to recognize your past complicity and understand the foundation from which it was born. But you must do so with self-compassion, nonjudgment and forgiveness. Release any guilt or shame you are holding onto. Accept yourself as you are, with love and gentleness, and begin recognizing the goddess within, starting right now. Know that you deserve total respect and acceptance. In this way, you can finally begin celebrating who you are, no matter what the rest of society tells you you should be.

3. *Action:* Here is a quick list of suggested actions you can take to begin accepting your present Being for the lovely creature she is. They may seem like small steps, but that is what any truly worthwhile process is about: small steps (some will be further expanded upon later):

- Stop watching ads that in any way suggest you are anything but perfect.
- When the diet ads come on television, hit the mute button or change the channel.
- Don't look at beauty magazines.
- Stay off the scale.
- Don't go on diets.
- Eliminate negative body talk.
- Feel compassion, not competition, for other women . . . and yourself.

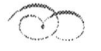

Personal Awareness— Who We Are

We ask ourselves, who am I to be brilliant, gorgeous, talented and fabulous?
Actually, who are you NOT to be?
—Marianne Williamson, *A Return to Love*, 1992

An essential piece of this process is assessing your beliefs and sorting out those that no longer work for you. Many of the beliefs we have about ourselves and who we are and can be in the world started when we were children and are often perpetuated by our continuing family dynamics. Some of those beliefs may have been created by us in order to survive some dysfunction in our childhood. Often, when those beliefs do help us survive, we become attached to them and take them with us into adulthood, thinking that they will do the same for us in the adult world. Sooner or later, we realize that most of those beliefs and coping mechanisms are not sufficient or helpful in the realm of grownup situations and relationships.

Finally coming to that realization can be quite traumatic, because it requires changing the way we see and change is always difficult, especially when it involves long-held and cherished beliefs. It is helpful to view those revelations with gratitude and celebration because they are the key to the door.

On the other side of that door is the limitless expanse of your life, filled with new options and the freedom to choose whichever of those options feel best suited to your adult Being.

Again, awareness is the key here. Most of our trauma and drama in this respect will come from the continuing attempts to make old solutions work in new situations. Once we are aware of what is happening, we are able to break free of those old thoughts and behaviors and find ones that support, encourage, and assist our growth and happiness.

The Power Tools in this chapter are a few suggestions for reaching this point of awareness. Different things work for different people, so see if any of these might assist you in identifying your belief systems. Whatever you choose to do, do it with compassion, nonjudgment and gentleness. Give yourself the same loving comfort and attention as you would a questioning child, for in many ways that is what you are in this process.

You might also wish to do this work with the assistance of a trusted, compassionate and supportive therapist. Often the objective view of a non-invested, nonjudgmental person can prove to be a powerful and necessary guide in your process. Don't be afraid to ask for help.

POWER TOOLS:

1. *Quiet your mind:*   One of the reasons you may not see how your belief systems are affecting your life is by not taking the time to focus your attention internally. This means finding time to yourself (knowing that you deserve it), away from other obligations, duties, engagements, demands. As often as you can manage it (the ideal would be at least once a day), go inside yourself. Take a bath, get a massage, meditate, do some yoga, or just sit and notice your breathing *(more on meditation and breathing in chapter 6)*. The goal is to calm your mind

and relax your body in order to open a connection with your inner self. Notice what feelings come up when you allow yourself to focus just on you. View it as a way of taking care of yourself and finding a path to greater joy in your life. Remember, if you never go inside, your won't be happy outside.

2. *Write Your Own "Herstory":* One way to help determine where your beliefs began, and thus find ways to change them if you choose to, is to write down your history. Find a quiet place where you can focus on yourself. Review your years of growing up: the family dynamics, relationships at school and with friends, events that made an impression on you. You don't have to share this with anyone; it is simply a tool for you to become more aware of where certain seeds were planted, how they took root, and why they have grown to be the seemingly unmovable trees they are today. Again, make no judgments about anything you remember or any feelings you have about it. Try to see things as they really were and what effect they had on you and how they might still be influencing your choices and assumptions in the world. Don't feel pressured to figure anything out at this point. Just concentrate on getting it down on paper and remembering with as much clarity as possible.

3. *Know Your body:* Become better acquainted with your body. Often we separate ourselves from our bodies, which results in us not taking care of them, not listening to them, not appreciating them. So, again, find a quiet place to be with yourself, calming your mind and focusing your thoughts. Think specifically about your body and allow yourself to notice how you are feeling and what assumptions and beliefs you hold. Do not judge any of it. This is just a beginning place to help you get a little more in touch with the Embodied You. *(See more in chapter 5.)*

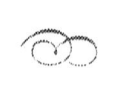

Mind Awareness—
What We Think

I will look for the thought that aligns me with Source, and I will live happily ever after.

—Abraham-Hicks, 2002

Belief systems come from many different places, but the most fundamental of them start rather early in our lives. The belief systems of our parents and those close to us tend to become ours, as well. Sometimes they are acquired in a very direct fashion (i.e., "Peas are good for you; ice cream is not.") Sometimes they are acquired by observation (i.e., although she said nothing out loud, you noticed her shame and anger when your mother stepped on the scale.)

Language is very powerful, and the words used to express concepts to us as children can be empowering and affirming or they can be wounding and damaging. Verbal and nonverbal indications to children that they are too much or too little or "too" anything can have devastating, long reaching consequences. As long as you are rigid about your belief systems, they will continue to rule your life and the self-fulfilling prophecy patterns will continue (i.e., if you believe no one will ever love you, they probably won't; if you believe everyone leaves you, they probably will). The challenge is to move beyond the belief system that creates the painful situation and create a new vision of what is possible. This requires a fundamental trust that you DO have the power to change what, up to this point, has been your reality.

The mind is a very powerful tool on the journey to body acceptance and unconditional self-love. Perception is reality. Therefore, what you think is what you live. If you think you are a victim or come from a place of hatred and misery, that is what you will bring more of into your life. If you live more from a place of power, self-love and joy, then those are the things that will become manifest in your life. What you "think" can literally mean the difference between living a life filled with happiness and abundance or allowing yourself to wallow in misery and lack. That being said, it makes sense that changing the way you see and think about things can change your reality. Pretty powerful stuff, huh?!

You are meant to live in joy and love. But before you can introduce these concepts at a spiritual and heart level, you first have to reframe as many of the past and present opposing thoughts as you can.

POWER TOOLS:

1. *If you wouldn't say it to someone else, then you aren't allowed to say it to yourself:* Your body is you, remember? She is connected to your mind and your heart. What you say to her you say to your soul. And that becomes the energy that is manifested into the Universe. Think about the things you say to yourself about yourself and your body. Ask yourself this question: "would I say this to someone else?" Would you turn to the woman next to you in the check out line or the next office and say to her, "those are the ugliest thighs I have ever seen? How can you even leave the house in the morning?" Of course you

wouldn't! And yet, you say such things to yourself all the time. Why do you think you deserve the kind of treatment that you would find cruel and rude when applied to others?

Stop all negative body talk. Stop all comments, judgments, and jokes about anyone's body. Notice when it happens, notice when others do it, and stop the thought as soon as you are aware of it. Don't judge yourself for it; don't begin blaming yourself for it. Just notice it and stop the thought. The most important thing here is to make sure that the first place you notice negative body talk is with yourself. You may find yourself having relatively few such judgments about others. But as you become aware of those things you say to yourself, you may be shocked at how cruel and heartless you are being. Negative body talk is self-abuse that keeps your body image and self-esteem anchored in the mud. It must stop. This may take a while to integrate, but be diligent. Soon you will find yourself noticing such thoughts right away, then find that you don't do it any more at all, and finally find yourself actually reframing them into positive, affirming things about your body.

2. *Throw away the scale:* One of the first ways you can eliminate negative body thoughts is to eliminate one of the most insidious sources: the scale. THROW IT AWAY! This may come as a surprise to some of you, but most women do not need to weigh themselves ever again, nonetheless every single day. A woman once said to me "It never occurred to me that I didn't have to submit myself to that daily torture." And that's just what it is! You wake up in the morning, you feel good, strong, healthy—then you step on the scale. Even one pound in the wrong direction can take that great good morning feeling and flush it down the toilet. That's a lot of power to invest in a couple pieces of metal and a

pinwheel of flying numbers. Please, don't let it happen to you ever, ever again.

3. *Define yourself:* As you proceed through the journey of being loving to your body, remember the following, from *Friendship with God* by Neale Donald Walsh: "EVERY ACT IS AN ACT OF SELF-DEFINITION." Sit with this concept, in meditation or in journaling or while you are washing the dishes: *every act is an act of self-definition.* Write it down; put it on the mirror. How do you wish to define yourself in the world? This phrase helped to further confirm my decision to inspire others to a place of celebration rather than anger. It was important to me to live my life through positive emotions rather than negative ones. Remember as you do this exercise that self-definition is an ongoing, continual, ever changing process, just like life. As you continue to grow and change and see things differently, who and how you want to be will change, as well. One affects the other. So stay open to the flexibility of this very dynamic process of self-definition.

4. *Identify your anger:* I heard somewhere that anger usually stems from one of three places: hurt, fear, or frustration. As you find yourself facing your anger in this process, identify it instead of denying it. Keep asking yourself questions until you come to some clarity about its source. Are you afraid of something? Did someone hurt you? Are you frustrated with certain things in your life? The more you can identify where your anger comes from, the sooner you can stop projecting it on yourself or others and work toward resolving it.

5. *Live "as if":* The importance of *attitude* in this process toward self-love and acceptance cannot be overemphasized. Once you begin ending the negative body talk (or negative ANY talk), once you begin balancing your thoughts more toward the positive, and once you begin defining yourself with each and every act in your day, then your attitude will change without effort. Affirmations are often quite helpful. One of my workshop participants said to me that she didn't like affirmations because they seemed to be untrue and she had promised herself she'd be honest. I told her that the affirmations aren't lies. It's just that we have forgotten their truth. It isn't a lie that we are beautiful, we have just forgotten that we are. So, what you are doing is living "as if" it were true until you open up the channel that lets you remember that it is.

Next time you are in a public place, take a few minutes to watch the people around you. See what their body language tells you. Notice how you perceive the woman who walks slouched over, head down, making no eye contact, perhaps with her arms clasped around her protectively in an effort to hide her body and become invisible. Now, notice how you perceive the woman walking tall, head up, inviting other people's gaze, smiling confidently, non-hesitant in her stride. This exercise isn't about making judgments about the lives of these women. The point is to notice how your "perception" of each woman changes. Now, notice how you present yourself to the world. Don't judge yourself. This is an awareness exercise to increase your clarity of self-attitudes you may not realize are there. Notice how your own feeling about yourself changes when you stand tall, shoulders back, facing the world head on. Remember, every act is an act of self-definition, including how you walk down the street. Our self-perception changes when our attitudes shift from embarrassment to pride, from fear to confidence, from hate to love. Once you do begin to remember the truth, people will notice the attitude change and will be drawn to your new contented, loving, proud, celebrated Being.

6. *It's not about you:* This notion comes from a book entitled *The Four Agreements,* written by don Miguel Ruiz. I have found it to be one of the most important ways in which I have changed my mind about the way I thought the world worked. The concept is simple: nothing anyone else does or says is about you. Everyone's reactions (including your own) are based on their own experiences, childhoods, beliefs in the world. They may be reacting to something you said or did, but what those reactions are or what they may say or project onto you is not about you. This is one of the ways in which we have let the cultural beauty standard effect us so deeply.

The societal messages about what is good and beautiful and acceptable are NOT ABOUT US. They are, indeed, about money and the perceptions of those who control it. We have taken these messages so to heart, believing that it means we, personally, are not good, beautiful or acceptable. That's a lie! Even when it's your mother who tells you that you aren't thin enough, it has nothing to do with you. It has to do with her own self-perceptions, the ideas she was brought up with, and the beliefs she has clung to. Maybe it's about her own lack of self-worth, which she finds intolerable, and therefore projects onto you. Your most important job in this situation is to not take her words personally.

This can be a difficult task with those you love, so practice with situations in which you are less invested. Say, the next Slim Fast commercial, or the person at the grocery store who gives you a look when you buy that bag of delicious two-bite brownies (my favorite), or the co-worker who, for no reason you know of, starts treating you like you are Lizzie Borden. Instead of becoming hurt and frustrated with the situation, instead of going into a defensive reaction, just say to yourself "it's not about me." You will notice immediately that instead of these types of events tying your gut in knots, you will be able to breeze by them with compassion and understanding. It's not about you.

You can practice this with things you say to yourself, as well. When you begin noticing your negative thoughts about your worth, say to yourself: who says so? You will likely find that it is not what you truly believe, but rather all those things that belong to your mother or your neighbor or society as a whole that you have taken in and believed were about you. Again, you need to bring yourself back to knowing: "it isn't about you." Only you can define who you are.

7. *Take responsibility for yourself:* In the same vein, remember that your reactions are only about you and not about whoever you are reacting to. Take responsibility for your actions and reactions. The example above about a co-worker actually occurred in my life. Although I work with this person every day, we have little in common and we are not really invested in each other's life. So, I was astonished at how her silent treatment could make me feel so bad. It felt almost as if my mother had said she didn't love me. Aha! This is when it became clear to me that my reactions weren't about my co-worker. She was just the trigger for my underlying issues about being lovable, being visible, being good enough. Her behavior made me feel unloved, invisible and below par. And as it dawned on me that it wasn't about her, it was about me, I began to feel so very much better. This revelation meant that I didn't have to wait for her to change. It meant I had control to change my perception and therefore change the experience.

Most people think that having someone else to blame for their bad feelings is a way to feel better. I find the opposite to be true. Once you are able to take responsibility for your own actions and reactions, there is always the possibility of things changing to a place you like better. When you rely on others to change, situations become hopeless. So, be grateful to those people who trigger you, because they help you to see the ways in which you have been hindering your own growth and happiness, and the ways in which you have given away your power. And once you can be grateful for something, it takes on an entirely different shape in your life, whether other people change or not.

8. *Create affirmations:* This is the time when affirmations are their most powerful and important. Changing your mind must be constantly reinforced with outside input, as well as inner work. So, make up those signs for the mirror, the refrigerator, the back of the bathroom door, even the ceiling over the bed. Put away all those negative thoughts, old ideas about not tooting your own horn (who else is going to do it, after all), and embarrassment at finally saying the truth. Be bold, use color. Make the affirmations short and sweet and easy to remember. Repeat them out loud and often! Here are just a few suggestions. Run with them!!

> I AM BEAUTIFUL.
>
> I AM GOOD ENOUGH
>
> EVERY ACT IS AN ACT OF SELF-DEFINITION.
>
> I BELIEVE IN LIVING IN JOY.
>
> I AM A PHENOMENAL WOMAN.
>
> I AM A GODDESS.
>
> IT'S NOT ABOUT ME!

Body Awareness— How We Feel

There are three billion women who don't look like supermodels, and only eight who do.

—The Body Shop, 1997

Now we move to the more tangible, which will eventually take you deeper inside your Divine space, for they are all connected and one cannot survive without the other. One of the best ways to combat the disconnection of mind/body/ spirit that this culture encourages is to become as aware of your body as possible. Acknowledging and caring for her, recognizing her as an integral part of your entire Being is a major first step. Without her, you would be just a poof of energy, unable to experience all the joys and delights of the physical realm. So ask yourself the following questions and focus on how it feels to be IN your body. Try journaling about each one so you really connect with your truth.

POWER TOOLS:

1. *How are you caring for your body?*

a. Have you accepted your body as a whole being?
This culture has a strong tendency to separate the body
from itself, to break it down into parts. Ads show only
belly buttons or legs or arms or hands—disembodied
pieces of meat. Often it is just the torso without a head.
There is no clearer statement that women are meant to be
"seen and not heard" than to show them without the
body part required to think or object. Don't dismember
your own body. Instead of finding fault with your thighs,
your stomach, or your hips, see your body as a whole
Being, with each part supporting the others, working
together quite admirably to keep you walking and lifting
and dancing and loving.

b. Are you listening to your body? Does she feel
like a part of you, and are you on speaking terms with
each other? She is very wise, but her voice can get
drowned out by the rest of the world. Listen to what she
is saying to you and express your gratitude to her for allowing you to live this physical life!

c. Can you breathe well? Breathing is a very important part of staying alive, as you know. Your body does
it all by herself. But do you find yourself breathing shal-
low, short, rapid breaths, instead of deep, slow, regular
breaths? Do you hold your breath in order to suck in
your belly? Finding ways to breathe fully and deeply will
help you find that connectedness between your mind/
body/spirit. Focused attention to your breathing is one
of the most healing and healthy things you can do for
yourself. *(See more in chapter 6.)*

d. Are you wearing clothes that fit? Clothes that fit
are an essential part of what makes you feel comfortable
in your body. Clothing that constricts your body or keeps

you from breathing well will only increase your feeling of discomfort with yourself. Throw or give away clothes that don't fit. Don't hold on to things because you think you might be that size again someday. If you are always looking at clothes that don't fit, you will continue to re-wind and play the "I'm not good enough" tapes in your head.

e. Do you pamper your body? Do you bathe her, lotion her, powder her, perfume her? Pampering your-self and your body in ways that feel soothing and soft or stimulating and tingly is a wonderful way to show your body that she is worth caring for. This can include full body massage, foot reflexology, energy balancing (through acupuncture or Reiki, for instance), or just sitting in the warmth of the sun (with your sunscreen on, of course). Self-pampering is a vital part of being an independent, self-loving person and an excellent way of taking care of that inner little girl who needs to feel your unconditional love.

f. Do you move in ways that feel good? Your body needs to be moved in order to keep working well. Find ways to move her that are enjoyable. The slow and sen-sual movements of yoga, the more aerobic pace of disco dancing, or just walking to the park or biking to the beach. And remember all those ways you naturally move your body everyday: stairs at work, chasing children, working the garden plot, vacuuming (that would be very irregular for me), and, of course, sex. Even breathing can be exercise if you do it right! Whatever you do, do it with joy and with the knowledge that you are caring for a pre-cious Being.

g. Do you feed her good food? Food is a book in it-self and will be discussed more in chapter 8. For now, suffice to say that healthy food is self-nurturing and so is the occasional delicacy. When you decide to have that delicacy, don't ruin the experience with guilt. Pay attention to your food and enjoy the deliciousness of every bite.

h. Do you visit a health practitioner? This is an important part of self-love, and often a difficult experience if you are fat or perceived as fat by yourself or others. Many women put off going to the doctor because of the dreaded "weighing in" process. I changed doctors years ago when the one I had wouldn't see me if I hadn't weighed in. None of my current primary caregivers require me to step on the scale. I never do. I also have chosen to do a good deal of alternative health care with a doctor of Chinese Medicine. This includes acupuncture, Reiki, healing touch, heat therapy, meditation, and herbal remedies. Western medicine certainly has its place, but alternative practitioners are often more interested in your whole life and in the least intrusive option available. Find a good balance between both medicinal worlds. Whatever you choose, find someone you trust, and, just as importantly, someone who trusts you and your own self-knowledge.

i. Do you give her enough rest? Enough water? Sleep and fluids are as vital as breathing to keeping you healthy and happy and energized. We rarely get enough rest and even more rarely enough water. Eight glasses of water a day sounds like a lot and feels that way when you start. But after a while, it will be so easy to do. Have a water bottle with you everywhere: at work, by the bed, on your bike, near the television. It's one of the best ways to keep your body cleaned out and your skin soft and supple.

Sleep needs vary with each person, so pay close attention to how much you require in order to feel rested and energetic. If you believe you are getting enough sleep and still feel tired, see your health-care giver. It could be as easily treatable as a dysfunctional thyroid gland, which is often misdiagnosed.

j. Do you tell her that you love her? Can you imagine never being told that you are loved by the person most important in your life? That's how your body feels when all you do is tell her what you hate about her. She needs to hear that she is loved as much as you need to hear it. And she's only going to get total unconditional love from one place: you!

k. Do you let others tell her that they love her? This is almost as important as telling her yourself. Quite often, we believe others don't love us when it is merely a projection of our own self-hatred. So, even when people tell us they love us, love our bodies, we don't allow that information in because we haven't managed to go there ourselves yet. Practice letting it in. It is the most glorious feeling to hear and believe someone when they say they adore your body . . . and you.

l. Do you tell her that she's beautiful? This is a lot about getting rid of negative body talk. Only say positive and wonderful things to your body. The more self-loving you are verbally, the more you will feel it inside. I read a story about a woman who, having been diagnosed with multiple sclerosis, decided that she wanted to feel unconditional love before she died. She knew that she was the only one who could do that. Every day, she sat in front of the mirror and told her body how beautiful she was, how much she loved her, how much she appreciated everything she did for her. Not only did this woman create the experience of unconditional love, she also healed her body. Her multiple sclerosis went into remission. Don't ever doubt the healing power of unconditional love and positive reinforcement; offer it to yourself and others often.

m. Do you let others tell her she is beautiful? Learn to take the compliments others give you. When you respond to a compliment with a negative or self-deprecating quip, you not only do yourself a disservice, but you dishonor the person giving the compliment. It has probably come from their most sincere feelings and to have it received with negativity can be very hurtful. So do both of you a favor—accept it with a smile. It's another example of living "as if." You may not believe the compliment now, but you will.

Try utilizing one of these three responses to compliments, using the third one as often as possible: "Thank you, I like hearing that"; "Thank you, tell me again"; "Thank you, I think so myself."

n. Do you accept touch and caressing with openness and joy? Okay, this one is mostly about sex. Not all touch is about sex, but when things turn sexually intimate most every woman's insecurities blossom. Sexual intimacy is the most vulnerable any two people physically get with each other, and the level of joy and pleasure you give and receive from the experience is often in direct relation with how much openness and acceptance of your body you have manifested. If you are thinking about whether or not your partner thinks your thighs are too big, you are not going to be focused on the incredible feeling of whatever he/she is doing to you. You sabotage your own pleasure. So, give them the benefit of the doubt and yourself the benefit of complete, orgasmic enjoyment of sensual and passionate touch.

o. Do you thank her for all that she gives you? Gratitude. The ultimate healing tool. Tell your body how much you appreciate all that she does, all the ways in which she makes it possible for you to be productive, active, and pleasured. It's amazing what she puts up with in this culture. It's time you gave her a big hug and a pat on the back.

Having seriously reflected on these questions, it's time to get even more intimate with your body. It is important to recognize that your body is your friend, not the enemy. Your body is the vessel in which you carry all of who you are. She houses your heart, your mind and your soul. She holds your love, your fear, your memories, your hopes, your passions and your dreams. She is your power, the fire in your belly. And it is that flame that lights your road to healing. The light is there, strong, secure, sure and everlasting. You just need to open the door and let it burn. Listening to your body is the first step to loving her. It's time for a conversation. So, when you are ready (and take your time; these things can bring up some very deep feelings), try the next tool.

2. *Dialogue with your body.* Find a quiet, safe place to sit, preferably before a mirror and preferably naked. Naked might be very difficult the first time, so do what's comfortable. Spend some time communing with your body. Breathe slowly, in and out, letting your belly expand with each in breath and collapse with each exhale; feel yourself breathing; settle into yourself. Watch yourself in the mirror; feel how you "fit" together; be aware of the thoughts that go through your head as you focus on your body. It is very important that you do this exercise with compassion, gentleness and nonjudgment.

Just for now, imagine your body as a separate being sitting across from you. She has heard everything you have thought. She knows how you feel about her. She wants to talk about it. Treat it as you would any conversation with someone close to you that you don't want to lose, but with whom you are feeling uncomfortable or irritated or annoyed or afraid or hurt or angry. Either of you may start. Be respectful, but deeply honest with how you feel about your body, and then listen as she tells you how it makes her feel and how she feels about you and what she needs.

Continue this process for as long as you can. If you begin getting uncomfortable, try to stay in that space, listening to what's being said. That discomfort is telling you that there is important information to be had, and it is vital to your healing that you allow yourself to feel it and bring it into the conversation. Be aware, as well, of how your body is physically feeling. Is she hurting, tense, tired, stiff, relaxed? It's all part of the conversation. Try to journal about your dialogue, if it helps. Such communications with your body are helpful throughout your process. As you progress on the mind and spirit level, it will have profound effects on the way your body feels and responds. And it will be very encouraging to you to track your progress as your conversations with her get more loving.

3. *Bodybuilding*: No, not that kind! This is about another wonderful way of connecting with your feelings about your body: sculpting. Any kind of clay will work, but I prefer the kind that is easy to mold and stays pliable until you bake it in the oven. Get colors that attract you, put on some fun music. You can even do it in a group with your friends. Now, just build a body. It can be the image of a goddess figure, your own body, the body of your favorite female role model, anything you want. But do it with love and mindfulness about the sacredness of the body and the ways you have already defined yourself to be, remembering what you have learned from your conversations with yourself. Do it with respect and honor and joy. HAVE FUN!

Spiritual Awareness— How We Love

Work like you don't need the money;
love like you've never been hurt;
dance like nobody's watching,
sing like nobody's listening;
live like heaven on earth.

—Author Unknown

Spiritual awareness is not about any particular religion or dogma or set of rules and instructions about a god or goddess separate from ourselves. It is about the Divine presence of the Universe within all of us. It's about your true essence. It's that piece of you that knows you are capable of unconditional self-love. From self-love flows all the goodness of the Universe. But because only a precious few of us are nurtured from childhood to believe we are worthy of love at all, self-love becomes an increasingly elusive state of the soul. When you are not moving in the world from a state of self-love, unfortunate and painful events often occur. So, your purpose—your mission, if you will—is to courageously explore your inner being and find that place of unconditional love that will allow you to manifest love, healing, joy, abundance, and gratitude in your life and in the world, instead of hatred, pain, misery, poverty, and anger.

POWER TOOLS:

1. *Live in the Moment:* Before you face the challenge of changing your mind and your heart and your spirit, it helps to practice the art of living in the "now." And in understanding that there is a difference between living *in* the now and living *for* the now. Living *for* the moment is probably the most unconscious way to live, because it is devoid of integrity or care about consequences. Living *in* the moment requires a great deal of consciousness, awareness and focus, for the simple reason that the choices you make now *do* have consequences, and choices should always be made with those consequences in mind. It's about considering options based on the information and wisdom you have garnered to that moment, without being a slave to the past or the future. It's about choosing to forgive the past (yours and everyone else's) and release your fear of the unknown future. The future becomes known only in the choices you make in the Now, and in this way you have the ability to create your own reality.

Each moment is perfect and you are perfect in it. You are on a journey that leads to growth and you choose in each moment how that growth will occur, but you are perfect within each moment. There is no space in the Now for anything but self-acceptance and love. "Growth" does not mean "better." The spiritual journey is about choices, ways you decide to live your life and define your Being in the world. Accepting your perfection in every moment is the key to making choices that will feed your soul and support your definition of integrity and self-love.

Willingness is also one of the keys to this process. By this I mean having a willingness to do more than try. Once you choose to "be" a certain way—once you begin your act of self-definition—it is reflected in every action and every choice you make from that moment on. Be willing to open the door to that level of responsibility, because the only way to *change* how you see is to be *responsible* for how you see.

2. *Create an Altar:* You may find it inspiring to have a special, sacred space in your living quarters that represents your spiritual essence; an altar of sorts, that contains items that speak of your life and have meaning on your deepest levels. Mine contains such things as a small representation of the ancient goddess; a small statue of a spirit of India; a picture of myself as a toddler (to remind myself of my precious perfection); a heart-shaped stone from a dear friend; a Tibetan singing bowl; a crystal from one of my spiritual teachers. Your altar should reflect who you are and give you comfort and a feeling of contentment. It's a space that can ground you and remind you that "you are not a human being having a spiritual experience; you are a spiritual Being having a human experience."

3. *Breathe:* There are many ways to calm your mind and access your true essence. But many people overlook the easiest and most useful tool: breathing. Most people don't think about breathing at all. Our bodies are miraculously able to take care of it with no conscious thought. But breathing is more than just the carrier of oxygen through the body. It can be a path to healing on all levels. Women especially tend to restrict the benefits of breath because bellies in this culture are supposed to be flat and unnoticeable, so we find ourselves breathing very shallowly, sucking in our stomachs, and stopping the flow of energy.

Nothing should restrict your breathing. Don't hold your breath. Don't suck in your belly. Don't wear tight clothes. Don't smoke. Nothing more than awareness of your breath is required to achieve great benefits. Once you consciously observe your breathing, you will find yourself naturally breathing deeper, slower and more deliberately.

There are many breathing techniques that are useful. For purposes of meditation you might wish to utilize some guidance until you are more practiced. Andrew Weil, M.D., has a wonderful set of tapes to teach proper healing breath. For now, all you need to know is that being conscious of your breathing is one of the most impactful power tools at your disposal. And you can do it anywhere, anytime. Begin by just *noticing* your breath. Put your hand on your belly and feel it expand with a full in-breath. Take breaths that are slow, deep and regular. Then you can move into more intentional breathing exercises useful in meditation, cleansing and reducing anxiety, to name a few.

4. *Have no expectations and an open heart:* One of the foundations for the spiritual journey is limiting your expectations of yourself and of others. This doesn't mean you think little of yourself. It merely means that you understand you are doing the best you can. Expecting perfection or expecting that people will do what you want them to do leads mostly to disappointment and frustration. But if you can greet yourself and others without such expectations *and* keep your heart open with compassion and love, you will find that you garner more love and appreciation than you ever could have "expected."

5. *Meditate:* Many people cringe at the suggestion that they begin the practice of meditating because they fear they are not "doing it right." I used to think that if I couldn't sit for hours on end "auhming" to the Universe without moving, then I was just a failure at meditation. I rarely utilized it. Then I removed all my restrictions on how meditation should be structured, and now I use it as a path to my soul, rather than just another way to beat myself up! So, I would like to demystify it a little.

* Remember, this is a tool to help you relax and release; it's not meant to be a torturous endurance test. Keeping your back aligned is important, but otherwise sit as and where you are most comfortable.

* You don't have to sit for hours. Start with five minutes. Stay with five minutes if it takes you where you want to go. I rarely sit for more than 20, and sometimes five is plenty.

* Got an itch? Scratch it! Need to stretch? Move. I find that removing the distractions is better than spending energy trying not to be distracted.

* Above all, meditation is a wonderful practice for the *no expectations and an open heart* tool. Expectations will only be another distraction. Do what you can to calm your mind, but don't expect to stop thinking completely. Sometimes what you end up thinking about it just what your meditation was meant to bring to light.

* With the help of your breath and a little non-judgmental patience, you can be relaxed and open to your inner voice.

With that in mind and all judgments released, let's try it. Be comfortable, back straight. Some subtle, soothing music can help minimize other distracting noises. Close your eyes, and begin taking deep, slow breaths, feeling your ribs and belly expand with each in-breath. Focus on your breathing in and out until you find a regular rhythm. Then follow the Relaxing Breath pattern for four full cycles.

The Relaxing Breath: Inhale through your nose quietly and exhale through your mouth noisily, exhaling with a kind of whoosh. Begin by exhaling through your mouth completely. Then inhale quietly through your nose to a count of four, hold your breath for a count of seven, and exhale through your mouth for a count of eight. Repeat that for a total of four breath cycles. The amount of time you spend doing the four breath cycles is not as important as the ratio of four, seven and eight. To reap the long-term benefits of the Relaxing Breath, do a minimum of four breath cycles twice a day, but never do more than eight breath cycles. This is a very powerful technique, and it has profound effects on physiology. . . .

—Andrew Weil, M.D.

Many things will come into your head. Try to return to a minimum of thought by focusing on your breath. Make no judgments about your thoughts; just recognize their presence and return to your breath. Every few breaths, try taking an extra few seconds to sit in the emptiness between the out breath and the next in breath. It is a very powerful place and is often helpful in taking you into a deeper relaxation. Keep breathing as the relaxation continues, releasing tension wherever you notice it. If you begin to feel emotionally uncomfortable or frustrated, continue breathing deeper and move into those feelings. This is exactly what meditation is for—to move you deeper into yourself, to expand your consciousness. This part will likely take the most practice. Again, don't judge yourself. The practice itself is it's own meditation.

Again, the most effective way to meditate is to have no expectations. Huge revelations or major emotional shifts probably won't happen in those five to twenty minutes. Meditation is a practice that, when done fairly regularly, serves the purpose of allowing an opening between your inner voice and your conscious mind. It is a cumulative effect. What you might find is that your revelations are occurring to you during your coffee break at work or while you are showering or just chatting with a friend. Even if you choose to not meditate in any structured way, practice the Relaxation Breath every day; it will in itself create a more balanced and healthy mind, body and heart space.

6. *Draw:* Often, after a meditation or when you begin having those "aha" moments of revelation, it is helpful to express them in some tangible way. It can help in understanding them and allows you to remember later what occurred for you. One of my favorite ways to do this is painting or drawing a Mandala,* which is a creation whose foundational structure is a circle. The circle is a universal symbol of wholeness and connection, and as such, it provides a powerful backdrop for the images that represent any visions which might occur during or after meditation. As with every life experience, the process of its creation is as important as the final product. Take your time. Close your eyes and "see" the feelings that arise, then transform them into colors and images and transfer that to paper. There may be shapes, there may be only colors, it might be abstract or realistic. Again, no judgments. Be thoughtful and aware and focused on this creation, for it reflects your belief about your place in the Universe. These images are as powerful as any affirmation, so put them up on the wall and reflect on them often.

7. *Journal:* Journaling is another common and powerful tool for recording your thoughts and visions. State the issue on paper, then just write a stream of consciousness

---

* "Mandala" is Sanskrit (an ancient language of India) for "whole world" or "healing circle." It represents the Universe and everything in it.

about it, whatever comes into your mind. The computer can often work well if you don't write as fast as your conscious stream is flowing.

However, do this with your monitor turned off, so as not to be distracted by typos or grammatical construction. Then you can just close your eyes and type whatever comes without any outside visual interruption.

Once again, do your journaling with no judgments on what it means, no worries of who it might offend. This is just for you, for your own understanding, your own awareness and clarity. This is not the time to hold back. It is a time to go deeper and closer to your own answers. It's always better to bring issues out into the open, into the light, whether you share them with others or not. No expectations and an open heart will be a key approach to this process.

8. *Other:* There are many other tools to reaching that quiet inner space that holds all the answers and secrets of your true self.

- Doing some sort of daily movement such as yoga or tai chi;

- getting a regular massage;

- visiting a Reiki Master or trained acupuncturist;

- consulting an oracle of divination, such as the Runes or tarot cards;

- watching something beyond beauty, such as a sunset or the amazing ways clouds form in the sky.

All things that focus your attention away from the chaos and drama of daily life are things that move you along the spiritual path.

Relationships

*Love is a force that focuses its light on the deepest shadowy
parts of ourselves.*

—Gay and Kathlyn Hendricks, *Conscious Loving,* 1990

Relationships. They are everywhere. They are inevitable. They
are everything. Friends, lovers, pets, co-workers, children, parents, siblings, the community, the Earth, the Universe. The
most important relationship, however, is with yourself.

This is a very strange concept to most women. We are social-
ized to take care of everyone else first and then ourselves . . .
maybe . . . if there's time before everyone else's demands resur-
face. We are expected to be the keepers of relationship in our
society. Without women to nurture the connection between
people, we would all be very isolated. But how can we maintain
this level of connection if we are not allowed to replenish ourselves? The quality of all the interactions we share with others is
affected and influenced by the quality of our own inner process.
If we are cut off from our soul, if we do not feel love for our
every cell, if we are not accepting of our own worth and divinity, then we will be cut off in our outer relationships, as well. We
will be unable to find true intimacy, or feel true love, or share
our true self. And we will take it on, feeling guilty and shamed
that we can't meet all those demands; just another way to not be
good enough.

POWER TOOLS:

1. *First you, then them.* The fact is, you have to take responsibility for your own fulfillment, your own satisfaction, your own happiness. You must begin to recognize that you have to be number one because you are the only one over whom you have control; and you are the only one who knows what you need. Then you can choose to give what you have to others in a way that continues to feed your energy, as well, rather than being sucked dry. It takes being centered in your Being, aware of your needs and wants in the world, and willing to endure the consequences of the people around you who feel betrayed at no longer being catered to. A friend of mine said that her thirteen-year-old daughter tells her mother's dates to be prepared to be number three. The daughter is number two, and the mother is number one. Unfortunately, most of the men don't really like the idea of not being first. Few people do. So, why should you?

First and foremost, be mindful of your relationship with yourself and your relationship with your body. You have been having dialogues with her, changing your perspective, giving her the benefit of the doubt. All of this is critical to having fulfilling relationships outside the sphere of your own skin. So keep practicing!

2. *Define what you want.* If you are unhappy with your relationships, it might be helpful to make a list of what you want them to be, as well as how you want yourself to be in them. Be specific, from the most practical to the most intimate to the most minute. List how they will feel about themselves; how they will feel about you; what they do in the world for work and for fun; what their spiritual philosophies are; how they feel about women in the world; what their politics are; how they will treat you; how they treat others; whether you can deal with snoring

or messiness or the toilet seat being up. This process allows you to continue defining yourself in ways that are positive and in harmony with your inner voice. It can also be extremely revealing if you are in a troubled relationship and can't figure out why. Relationships are very complex and extremely personal to the people involved. Don't let yourself be fooled into thinking that you must want what the world says you must want. Want what YOU want.

3. *Show Up.* A friend once said to me when I was whining about my relationship at the time, "well, what do you expect: you get into a relationship and then you don't show up." What she meant was that once in relationship, I stopped being me and became who I thought my partner wanted me to be instead. The lesson was that I need to connect with my true essence and then make sure she SHOWS UP! Don't let anyone tell you that you aren't good enough. And certainly don't say it to yourself—ever, ever again. *Every act is an act of self-definition* is at work again here. In relationships most of all, it is vitally important to remain mindful of who and how you wish to BE. It may be a fluctuating thing, but staying aware of your inner truth each moment will help you flow with the impermanence of life and the sometimes roller coaster relationship ride. As Dolly Parton says, "figure out who you are and then do it on purpose!" You will find yourself happier with yourself and attracting more and more relationships that fulfill your desires.

4. *Be naked often.* Being naked is wonderful and freeing. Most women tell me that, if it weren't for the fact that they hate their bodies, they would be naked waaay more often. DO IT. You can't be comfortable being naked with someone else if you aren't comfortable being naked alone. Practice feeling the freedom of letting your body

breathe. Pass mirrors, look at your body, and tell her she's beautiful.

5. *Sex is not the enemy*: We are constantly reminded that a woman's sexual identity is inextricably tied to her body; so much so, that people often don't notice the sensuality of our voices or the desirability of our warmth and personalities or the attractiveness of our souls. If we don't have big enough breasts, a small enough waist, long enough legs . . . why look further? The real kicker is that this is not what always actually happens in the world. There *are* men and women out there who don't completely buy the beauty standard brainwashing. But it doesn't matter what *actually* happens; it's what we *believe* will happen, what we are *told* will happen that motivates and/or paralyzes us. Here's the paradox: we spend so much time and energy trying to look the way we are told to look and behave the way we are told to behave, that we don't have the time or energy to just be and appreciate ourselves. This usually means that others see us most often in a state of self-dissatisfaction, which doesn't leave much room for seeing us as sensual, sexy, warm or soulful. If we don't see ourselves that way, how can they?

Even those eight women in the world who look like supermodels have fears about sex and intimacy. So it's no surprise that the three billion rest of us would, as well. But, if you are also fat, it becomes more than scary; it becomes terrifying—and sometimes impossible. Many women already don't feel worthy of attention and love, even in the most benign of situations. It very often keeps us from making eye contact with strangers on the street, to say nothing of being naked with someone in whom we have a vested interest.

Many women use sex as a source of instant gratification; as a way to feel loved, even if just for a moment.

But trying to fill an inside emptiness from an outside source never provides any lasting satisfaction. In addition to the tangible potential for physical disaster (unwanted pregnancy, sexually transmitted diseases), there is the inevitable damage to our spirit, damage that can be difficult to repair. The first step to making sex a sacred experience is to honor yourself and your body enough to go to that level of intimacy only with people with whom you have already established a mutual respect. Then, if and when the time arrives to move into a clothes-optional situation, you need to look for a way to rise above the physical. In passionate circumstances, your soul should lead the way—not your fat cells.

Another way to be ready for those intimate occasions is to create a few of them for yourself when you are alone. Buy yourself a really good electric vibrator and any other sex toys you feel comfortable about. Hunt down some erotic prose or poetry or write your own. Create a romantic, sensual atmosphere in your bedroom, with candlelight, soft music, clean soft sheets, slinky lingerie, whatever makes you feel warm and sexy. Then, make love to yourself. Touch yourself, move your body, make noise, stretch the foreplay or go right for orgasm. But pay attention to how your body feels and what you like. You deserve to be pleased when you are making love and there's no better way to know how to make that happen than to do it for yourself. This will be one less thing you have to think about when the time comes. It also makes for great bed talk!

The most important thing is to remember that sex is really very little about the body and very much about attitude and soulfulness and self-love. There is nothing more sensual than someone who loves her body and knows how to accept pleasure, thereby giving pleasure to her partner, as well. Trust me, if you've gotten far enough to have this person between your thighs, you can bet they aren't thinking about how big they are. And neither should you!

6. *Women united*: As you begin defining how you wish to be in intimate relationships, you will find that many of those qualities are important in your relationships with friends, family and community, as well. Mutuality, respect, presence, attention, acknowledgment, integrity, compassion, love. These are factors that should be standard practice in all relationships, regardless of level of physical intimacy. Pay particular attention to how you manifest these qualities with other women. Even though this culture has an insidious way of turning us against each other, what we really desire is support, comfort, understanding and unity. And we are responsible for making that happen. Take good care of your female friendships and respect all women, understanding that you all have something in common.

7. *Pamper your divine self*: Remember to give time and attention and energy to your relationship with the presence of the Divine in your life, in whatever form that takes. You are a sacred Being. The more you can connect with that reality, the more free and joyous your relationships will be.

Health

*Over and over, I'm impressed by the power of breath and its
ability to correct specific health problems and promote our
general well-being.*

—Andrew Weil, MD, 1999

I found this great synonym for "healthful" in the Webster's
Thesaurus: "salubrious." I love this word because it sounds full
and robust and joyful and a little lustful—all the things healthful should be. But the whole idea of health has garnered a pretty
suspicious reputation with women and fat people, because it is
used as a scare tactic. It's a weapon, and one that's wielded
rather effectively. No, I'm not a doctor, and yes, there are some
people who are more susceptible to illness because of their
weight. This isn't about ignoring your health care giver. It's
about educating both her and yourself, and taking control of
your body and how she is treated. It is also about recognizing
that some of the perceived ill-effects of being fat are not physical, but may actually be connected to how poorly fat people are
treated in this culture and the emotional stress it can cause.

Perhaps out of fear that you might be catching on to the real
reason for keeping you dissatisfied with yourself (i.e., greed), the
media brokers want you to think that they have shifted their
emphasis from "beauty" to "health." But the fact is that the

ideas of health and beauty in this culture are irrevocably married to each other. Thin means healthy, fat means sick; young means healthy, old means sick. The medical profession has made the same mistake as society at large by making blanket statements about fat and lumping all people together in their assessments. I am definitely considered fat in this country, but my health care givers—both traditional and alternative—have declared me quite salubrious. There is no reason for your size to be used as a baseline for assumptions about your health.

We are also told that being fat *creates* illness: high blood pressure, heart disease, even cancer. The "experts" assume that fat people are unhappy or unhealthy because of their fat. Has it ever occurred to anyone that some of our illness might be caused by the internalization of the shame we experience by living in a thin-obsessed society? It certainly is the basis for the life-threatening illness of eating disorders. In the Fiji Islands, where there is no cultural obsession with thinness, eating disorders were very rare. However, the incidents of eating disorders quadrupled once the Fiji population began receiving American television shows that only portray small bodied women. This phenomenon among the Fiji women has nothing to do with health and everything to do with image.

Honor your body and respect her needs. Listen to what she wants. Read labels to see about whether things are organic or contain partially hydrogenated anything or other things that could actually harm you. Don't obsessively count calorie intake or only allow yourself certain foods at certain times of the day. Diets that work on the premise of "rewarding" you for your ability to deprive yourself set you up to feel like a failure if you don't follow the rules. This does not promote self-care, it perpetuates self-loathing.

Almost all diets are about self-loathing. A *change* in your diet, i.e., deciding to eat vegetables on a more regular basis, switching to organic yogurt, trading in whole milk for soy milk, is different than *being on* a diet. The goal of *being on* a diet is losing

weight; a *change* in your diet is made for the long-term and becomes part of your nutritional, self-loving self-care. And even
then, those ideas about how you want to eat should be flexible.

This society tends to place "good" and "bad" judgments on
everything we eat. Vegetables are good and chocolate is bad; tofu
is good, ice cream is bad. Ever notice that there are far more
"bad" foods for fat people than for thin people? Some people have
the impression that ice cream sundaes are somehow healthier if
you are thin. The fact is that sugar has just as many empty calories
whether you weigh 90 pounds or 290 pounds. Ads that say things
like "It tastes naughty, but it's not," or "Bad never tasted so
good" only increase the guilt and shame when you dare to eat for
pleasure. Judging foods as good or bad eventually translates into
judging people who eat them as good or bad.

There is a difference between *will power* and *self-care*. Will
power denotes deprivation and guilt; self-care is about self-love
and integrity. As long as everything you do with and put into
and say to your body is about self-care and self-love, then go for
it. But if it's about proving you have control in your life or proving you have will power and are capable of depriving yourself
(and thus living up to that which the culture demands from
you), then there are emotional elements at work that need to be
addressed. Feel good about putting healthy things in your body
because you know that internally your body is working better
and you will be able to live a longer and freer life. It feels good
to know that you are capable of caring for yourself with love and
nurturance and not out of some misguided, perverse sense of
obligation the culture has imposed on you.

As in all things, it is a question of balance. This is about you
feeling good about how you are in the world, not who someone
tells you to be. It's about finding your own natural weight and
size and shape and loving it every step of the way. So, when you
choose to eat anything, be it sautéed zucchini or a dark chocolate truffle, do it with passion and enjoyment, not with guilt.
You want your body to be as healthy as possible for as long as she

lasts. But being healthy isn't just about what you put in your body, but how you feel about putting it in your body. It is not healthy to eat and then feel guilty, or *not* eat and then feel deprived. Healthy eating in a shame-free environment is a glorious way of increasing the happiness of whatever years we have.

There are also myriad other opportunities out there for making your body different that have nothing to do with what you eat. You are not just a body, and your body is not just "parts." You are a whole, integrated, connected being, with a heart, a mind and a soul. You are who you are for a reason. To hack at it, dissect it, suction or staple it somehow seems to dishonor the original unique creation that is you. However, you may still want to change your body, so, let's compromise: at least be sure that you are doing it not because of the harassment from a misogynist, economically driven society, not out of shame, not out of self-hatred. Such serious decisions should be made only out of your truth, your self-knowledge, your essence. And should you make the decision to change your body, take time, think again, feel again, search again for the absolute truth of what you are doing. Only then does changing your body emanate from our integrity, as all things must.

POWER TOOLS:

1. *Envision health*: First and foremost, believe that you deserve a healthy body, regardless of its size or age, and stop spending valuable energy worrying about what might happen. The more thought you place on being sick, the more likely you will be to get sick. Always envision yourself as healthy and vibrant and energetic.

2. *Care of your body*:

   a. **Movement**: Move your body in ways that feed your soul. Movement is imperative to a strong, flexible body and vital, productive organs. But many people aren't movement motivated, and the idea of "exercise" often causes negative emotions about competition, fear of failure, injury. For fat people, it can also evoke feelings of embarrassment and humiliation. But instead of avoiding movement, find something that you love to do and don't call it "exercise." Call it "recreation" or "a date with your body," anything that represents fun and not duty. Walk, swim, bicycle, dance, trampoline, hike, do yoga, lift weights, kayak, play tennis, golf, martial arts, belly dance. The options are endless. The only trick is giving yourself permission to try them until you find what you love, with no pressure, no competition, no fears of failure, no humiliation. Do what feels good and makes you happy.

You will likely find that movement works on an emotional and spiritual level, as well. Yoga can connect you to your quiet inner space; belly dance can connect you to your lost female empowerment; tai chi or martial arts can connect you to your feeling of physical and mental power. Find what works for you on all levels.

b. Food: Remember that eating is a natural form of nurturing, comfort, and self-care, not to mention survival, and should never be about deprivation and shame. Generally speaking, eat healthy foods. But read up a little, because there is a lot of misinformation out there.[*] I deplore the concept of deprivation and strongly support the use of fresh, organic, free-range foods (when possible). Eating healthy does not mean eating boring. Organic foods actually taste better. Soy milk works well on cereals and as a substitute in sauces. I eat more vegetables, make fruit smoothies (really good in the summer), eat Basmati or brown rice instead of white, and have darker and denser breads, with organic butter. However, I also

---

[*] I recommend *Eating Well for Optimum Health,* by Andrew Weil, M.D.

love Paul Newman's Butter Boom microwave popcorn and adore these little homemade brownies I find at the grocery store. It's about balance, not deprivation.

c. **Diets**. Most diets are unhealthy in the long run. Any food program that works on a system of deprivation and reward will not have a lasting positive effect in your life. Find a way of eating that feeds your physical hunger, satisfies the pleasure of your taste buds, doesn't leave you feeling deprived or guilty, and promotes a strong, well-balanced, energetic body, which does not necessarily mean a "thin" body. Don't compare yourself with others . . . not your size or the way you choose to eat. Everyone's body and health are unique and need to be treated with respect and focus. Choices about your eating should be based on self-love, self-care, awareness and respect for your individual needs and desires.

d. **Care-giver**: Find a health care giver who honors you as the person responsible for your own health. Take time to decide what you truly need in this relationship, which may include Western medicine, as well as other alternative methodologies. Whomever you choose, make sure they respect your choices regarding your care and trust your knowledge of your body and the state of your well-being. Trust is an absolute necessity in this relationship, so don't settle for anything else. You should always feel empowered, respected, and in charge when dealing with your health care givers.

3. *Care of your mind*: A healthy mind is vital to overall well-being. How well you have learned to cope with the ways of the earth-plane world will have a huge influence on how healthy and fulfilled your life is, on all levels. In the process of learning to wander through the labyrinth of being a physical being, the power of thought has become absolutely clear.

a. **The law of attraction**. The law of attraction is basically this: that which you focus on is what you get. If you are thinking mostly negative thoughts, that is what will likely be your experience; if you are thinking mostly positive thoughts, then your experience will be largely positive. To determine whether a thought is negative or positive, notice how you *feel*. If you feel good about what you are thinking, then those thoughts are in harmony with the positive aspects you wish to create. If you feel bad about your thoughts, you are inviting negativity into your life. Along with noticing whether your thoughts feel good or bad, remember to focus on believing that you deserve all the wonderful things you think about. This opens up the vibrational space necessary for them to flow into your life. Being filled with self-doubt and low self-esteem (which feels bad) blocks the goodness of the Universe from flowing to you, or at least slows it down. Being self-confident and self-loving (which feels good) lets in the innate goodness you deserve. Practice reframing those tapes in your head that cast you in a negative light and replace them with positive, uplifting, self-loving thoughts.

b. **Don't take it personally**. As I mentioned earlier, a favorite book of mine is *The Four Agreements,* by don Miguel Ruiz. The concept is that, from birth and sometimes before, we are taught our beliefs by others, and by living according to those beliefs, we have tacitly agreed to their truth. Ruiz believes there are only four agreements necessary to live a joyous, integrous and spiritually fulfilling life. They are:

(1) Be impeccable with your word.

(2) Don't take anything personally.

(3) Don't Make assumptions.

(4) Always do your best.

These four agreements can be very helpful, not only in navigating through the external world, but in training your mind to think differently about yourself. Here's how I see them relating to your body image: (1) *Being impeccable with your word* means that there can be no more negative body talk or badmouthing about your body or yourself; (2) *Not taking anything personally* is knowing that when other people say things that hurt you, whatever they say is not about you, it is about them, and comes from their own fears and past experiences; and knowing that the same is true about you, and taking responsibility for what is yours; (3) *Not making assumptions* is perfect for helping you open up to those people who show you attention and say they love you. So often your own self-hatred closes you off to those who do love you because you assume that they couldn't possibly be telling you the truth; and (4) *Always do your best*, at all things, because it is about your integrity and about being your true self in the world. This agreement also is about not regretting your actions or second guessing your decisions. If you try your best and look back without regret, you eliminate the temptation to punish yourself for your past perceived failures.

4. *Care of your spirit*: The health of your body and mind, of course, is intimately and undeniably tied to the health of your spirit, and vice versa. What affects one affects the other. Having a spiritual awakening can have a profound effect on how you think and treat your body; changing the chatter in your head can be extremely uplifting to your spirit and result in new self-nurturing practices toward your body; strong bodies, filled with nourishing and satisfying food, can't help but create loving thoughts and joyful spirits. Therefore, taking the time and space to go within is of paramount importance to the health equation. Seek out or create a practice that

allows quiet time so you can hear that inner voice of truth, that voice that knows your true essence and holds the strength to empower you in every way. This practice can include meditation, making music, creating art, cooking, gardening, writing, communing with nature. Again, the options are limitless. Choose those things that allow you to connect with your deepest and highest self, that allow you to communicate with the Divine that is within you, creating the foundation to be strong and complete in the external world.

At the risk of repeating myself, I once again urge you to pay more attention to your breathing. The breath is the most commonly used vehicle for communicating with your inner voice, your spirit. Deep, slow, mindful breathing can have far reaching affects on your body, mind and spirit. The more unrestricted your breath, the more freely and fully it flows where it is needed. Certain methods of breathing can not only calm and quiet your mind, but actually promote physical healing. Breathing exercises are often recommended for people suffering from anxiety and nervousness. It helps focus your thoughts and still the chaos. There is a reason why when people are upset, anxious, scared, or excited, the first thing most people will say to them is "breathe."

Finally, I would highly recommend reading anything by Christiane Northrup, M.D., author of, among other things, "Women's Bodies, Women's Wisdom," and "The Wisdom of Menopause." Check out her books and her website at www.drnorthrup.com.

Role Modeling

There's no better time than now to help our daughters,
young and growing, learn to love their bodies.

—"Love Thyself" book review of
101 Ways to Help Your Daughter Love Her Body
(2001, www.webheights.net/lovethyself/books.htm)

Everyone needs someone to look up to and identify with; someone who looks like you, tells the same truth, leads the kind of life you want to emulate, shows you that you are accepted and not alone. People, especially children, learn a great deal about themselves through other people. This is why mentoring programs have proven so successful. Diversity in advertising has come a long way in recent years. There are now more ethnic groups, more races, more women represented in the media than ever before. Most everyone can read magazines, watch television ads, go to the movies and see someone they can relate to in a positive, affirming manner. Everyone, that is, except fat people, especially fat women. Rarely are fat women in a prominent role in either entertainment or advertising—unless they are needed to carry the joke.

POWER TOOLS:

1. *Seek out true role models.* There are a few women in Hollywood who defy the "norm": Tyne Daly, Kathy Bates, Kathy Nijimy, Oprah Winfrey, Rosie O'Donnell, Camryn Manheim, Melissa McCarthy (The Gilmore Girls). Oprah and Rosie could be having an enormous influence in this regard. They both have everything anyone could ask for: fame, power, influence, money, adoration both personally and professionally. And still, they are both on the constant quest for a smaller body. I am grateful to Oprah for bringing the concept of spirit and self-awareness into the mass consciousness; I am grateful to Rosie for her incredible generosity of money and time to causes supporting women and children. I can empathize that, with all they have, they still are victims of the patriarchal culture and unable to use their incredible good fortune to set an example of how inconsequential body image should be.

Camryn Manheim, however, is another story. She is a true fat activist, who has been publicly outspoken about the discrimination and oppression of fat people, especially women, in this culture. When she won the Emmy award, she ended her speech with "This is for all the fat girls!" She has written a best selling book entitled *Wake Up, I'm Fat!* and did a great television movie called "Kiss My Act" (in which she is warm and funny and gets the guy!). There is no one I respect more in this regard, and she gets my Role Model of the Century award.

Seek out role models in your own life who are positive, strong, self-loving women, with attitude and spirit and sass. More importantly, be one yourself.

2. *Read affirming, joyful books.* Look for books that support who you are and tell affirming stories about women of all sizes. In addition to Camryn's book, I also

highly recommend a novel by Jennifer Weiner entitled *Good in Bed* (a sweet and funny story of a plus-sized journalist, her clueless ex-boyfriend, and her marvelous journey through the maze to self-acceptance), and *Kiss My Tiara* by Susan Jane Gilman (an outrageous and funny kick-ass, action-oriented approach to the issues women face, from body to men to family to work).

3. *Throw away "beauty" magazines.* As noted earlier, beauty magazines can destroy a woman's self-esteem in less than three minutes. Don't put yourself through this torture. Unfortunately, magazines aimed at women size 12 and over, like *Radiance* and *Mode,* have not survived. Another sign of the times. However, look for *Sage Woman*, which celebrates the goddess spirituality and speaks to your deep, inner strength.

4. *Treat your children well.* Role models are important for women because women become the role models for little girls and adolescents. There is no more important job for women today than to set a good example of strength, self-love and acceptance for their daughters and other girls (and boys) in their lives. Adolescents are our most fragile population. Women used to report that body image distortion and eating disorders started in college. But that has changed drastically. Today it has been found that 60% of fourth grade girls are on a diet. That's age 10, the age when girls' bodies are changing drastically in the normal process of growing into a woman. This growth should proceed unimpeded. It should be supported and revered. Girls should be feeling like the transition into womanhood is a positive and celebratory experience, to be honored and blessed.

Instead, they are told that they are getting fat (i.e., no longer looking like a boy) and that they must begin to restrict their activities (i.e., must become more "ladylike"). It soon begins to crystallize for these young girls that physical appearance and proper behavior must be the ways to happiness. Controlling their food intake, depriving themselves, becoming obsessed with their weight and their looks are all supported as "good girl" behavior, necessary to stave off the horrors of having a round, full, curvaceous body—a woman's body. Dieting can be extremely damaging at any age, but when a body is not yet fully developed, that damage can be irreversible and even fatal.

5. *Communicate with your daughters.* "Do as I say, not as I do" will NOT DO in the area of body image and self-acceptance. You cannot tell a girl that she is beautiful and perfect just the way she is and then go into a tailspin when you step on the scale yourself. Girls will see your distress and quickly believe that putting on weight is definitely not okay no matter what we may say to them.

Take specific, intentional time to speak with your daughter about her concerns and questions about her body, explaining that the roundness, higher body fat, and larger hips and thighs are a natural part of being female; let her know what she might expect in the patriarchal media world and help her find ways to not take it personally; support the development of her innate intuition and self-knowing; encourage healthy eating without deprivation or judgment; discourage dieting of any sort; support a strong healthy image of women's bodies; help her to find her own natural body size and shape, whether it be slender or not; teach her that true beauty is inside and comes from an attitude of strong self-esteem, self-respect and self-love. Create for her an environment that is non-judgmental, shame free, and filled with unconditional love.

Two books I would recommend for those involved with young girls are *Reviving Ophelia: Saving the selves of adolescent girls* (Pipher) and *101 Ways to Help Your*

Daughter Love Her Body, (Rehr and Richardson). *Reviving Ophelia* will give you a hard and perhaps surprising look at the expectations, dangers and choices young females face in this society and what parents can do to become aware of and active in this process. *101 Ways* is a practical list of things parents can do to help their daughters combat the social and peer pressures they might be facing, and help them see that there are other options than hating/changing/starving their bodies.

6. ***Communicate with your sons.*** Boys need the very same level of rolemodeling. Growing up with women who are obsessed with their weight and their appearance only serves to reinforce what the media is saying about what girls should look like. Boys soon learn in this society to believe that there is something wrong with fat girls and that to be seen with them means there is something wrong with them, as well. Girls who deviate from the ideal "look" are likely to not be seen for their other qualities, since the physical image is what attracts interaction. Teach your sons about self-respect and self-love and how to honor girls similarly. If they can find their own true selves, they will be more likely to appreciate it in women.

7. *Start young.* You must not wait until girls are teenagers for this role modeling to begin. A woman recently told me that she is already concerned for her two-year-old daughter because she is plump and her three-year-old cousin is tall and lanky. The family is already beginning to compare their body types. This woman wants nothing more than to keep her daughter from the turmoil of such comparisons. There is little she can do to shield her daughter from the social onslaught of beauty messages, but she can model for her daughter a woman who is strong, confident, self-loving and accepting of her body. She can be there to discuss these issues when her daughter comes home crying about

some senseless, cruel remark at school. She can discuss with her family that making comparisons between the cousins is not an appropriate way to support and encourage self-confidence in either of them. The negative messages begin early, and so must the positive counter-measures.

8. *Speak up, speak out.* Another part of role modeling is to speak out when you see or hear other people doing or saying things to girls that make them feel badly about how they look or who they are. When told by a friend that her twelve-year-old niece was being constantly berated by her mother about her weight and what she ate, I strongly suggested that she say something to her sister-in-law. Saving that child from the probability of years of continuing that cycle, possibly resulting in a damaging and potentially deadly eating disorder, is far more important than whether or not the well-intentioned but ill-informed mother is insulted by the intervention. Be bold enough to make people aware and more educated about their fears of fat and the devastating effect those fears have on our children—and, therefore, on us all.

For yourself and your daughters and your sons—indeed for all future generations—you must change the way *you* see, so that what *they* see is a way to be self-loving, accepting and honoring of the transformations their bodies are undergoing.

Healing Ourselves

*Healing involves moving toward wholeness. Healing gently
dissolves limiting thoughts and moves us toward acceptance
of all aspects of ourselves.*

—Barnett and Chambers,
Reiki Energy Medicine, 1996

W omen in this society are expected to nurture everyone
else before themselves. No wonder we burn out. We are not
taught how to take care of ourselves first. No one tells us that
unless we take care of ourselves first, there will be little or
nothing to give anyone else. And when we finally do burn
out, we often get blamed for either the absence of our
nurturance or at the very least the lack of quality it contains.
Giving and receiving are of equal importance and should be
assigned equal validity, no matter what your gender or status
in the world. We must take time—quality time—to replenish
our energy at the deepest levels or soon we will find ourselves
without any. Because society trains us to do otherwise, we
must take control and do this for ourselves.

This journey will require no small amount of reframing the
old beliefs that are holding you back and keeping you from re-
alizing your full potential. The way to accomplish this is by
changing our perspective, of both ourselves and the world. You,

of course, must start with changing the way you see yourself. No real, lasting change can be accomplished by beginning externally. The internal work is essential.

POWER TOOLS:

1. *Healing the mind*

a. Self-visualization

See your body as a vehicle. She needs to be given attention, be kept well fed with properly balanced fuel, have regular check-ups, be rubbed down on occasion, be kept safe from bumps and nicks, be well oiled to move efficiently and painlessly, and accessorized occasionally in order to show off her personality. Vehicles come in all shapes, sizes, colors, and ages. Some run smoother than others; some may have been in a few more accidents or lived in a rougher neighborhood than others; some are more well fed; some get used more than others. How well they work for the time they are needed depends on how well cared for they are. And that's the owner's responsibility.

See your body as your child. She counts on you to take care of her and love her unconditionally so she can feel good about herself and present herself with pride and self-love. She is very loyal and will always love you. However, she will not function well if abused, verbally or physically. She will become beaten down and miserable and depressed and unhappy. She may even become ill in order to get your attention. She needs you to be her protector and her champion. She needs you to shield her from outside abuse and intolerance. If she feels fully and unconditionally accepted by you, it will matter a lot less what anyone outside says or does. She can face the outside intolerance if she knows she is safe with you.

See your body as a temple. Your body is a holy place. She deserves to be viewed and treated in a sacred manner, to be spoken to with reverence, to be worshiped as the source of your breath, your fire, your power, your life blood. Indeed, it is your body that houses your soul and provides the sanctuary in which you integrate your whole being in this physical reality, grounding you so you may proceed with your life's mission. Your body is a holy place.

Remember that your body is you. She deserves to be treated with love and respect and honor, just as you do; to be celebrated for who she is right this minute and for the space she claims in the world. Treat her well, dress her up, display her with pride, and move through the world from a place of pure authenticity.

b. Self-affirmation. It is time to return once again to those self-definitions we have been talking about. Many of us have difficulty believing that we actually are who we want to be. We know it at some level; we feel it as true. But society tells us not to be vain or self-important, so we hide ourselves away, wasting all that beauty and wonder. One of the most important ways to keep aware of your inherent magnificence is to write out affirmations. It is a very powerful way of retraining your mind and heart to believe the truth instead of the lies you have been told.

Affirmations can come in many forms: bumper stickers, buttons, phrases in books, greeting cards. There are many inspiring writings out there that speak to the basic human condition. You can generalize about a lot of this information and about how we can "all" find our way through it. But the actual "way" to find the way through is going to be different for everyone. So, the most powerful affirmations are those which you create yourself about your own human condition. Affirmations should

speak to who you are, how you got here, who you want
to be, and where you want to go.

Look closely at the quality you wish to believe (and
already know the truth of at some level), and reduce it to
its most succinct expression. Some of those for me have
been "no expectations and an open heart," "divine vis-
ibility," "just say yes," and, of course, "celebrate your
body." All of these have been born from a state of discomfort that arose when I forgot that I am already
worthy, beautiful, and perfect. Affirmations are just re-
minders of who you are.

Make a commitment to do this work in your life: pon-
der what triggers you, process what it means for you,
what you want to change, how you can make that happen, and how you can create your own definitions of who
you want to be in the world, based on your true essence.
This process is about healing yourself, and you are the
only one who knows what that requires.

c. **Create your own reality.** As I have mentioned,
the laws of the Universe tell us that what you focus on
is what you will attract into your life. If you are focused
on the lack of something in your life, you will attract
more lack. If you are focused on the abundance in your
life, you will attract more abundance. It sounds pretty
simple, but it takes awareness and a lot of practice. How
you are experiencing your life is a direct reflection of the
balance of your positive and negative thoughts. If what
you are thinking about makes you feel good, then you
are in harmony with your inner intentions. If what you
are thinking about makes you feel bad, then you are not
in harmony and will attract that which you don't really
want. Relating this theory specifically to your body: if
you are unhappy with your body, if you hate your body,
if you believe that no one could love your body or you,
then you are undoubtedly feeling bad. In this frame of

mind, you will likely attract more self-hatred, more un-happiness, and more people who berate your body. However, if you are self-loving, happy, proud and confident about your body and your worth in the world, then you will undoubtedly attract more happiness, more love, and many people who are also proud and confident, and who are attracted to that in you. Dieting, for instance, is about lack. This is not in harmony with your higher good. Self-care, however, is about abundance and self-love and will result in more of the same.

This theory about the laws of the Universe goes hand-in-hand with self-definition. When you can relate your ideas of who you are with how it makes you feel, you will have little trouble defining yourself in the world in ways that bring you harmony and abundance and wholeness.

2. *Healing the heart.* Healing happens on multiple levels. Affirmations are an excellent way to retrain your mind to think and perceive differently. But you must also heal your heart and this is often a more difficult task. The two most powerful tools in this heart-healing process are gratitude and forgiveness.

a. **Be grateful**. In Neale Donald Walsch's *Friendship with God*, he states that "gratitude is the fastest form of healing." This is another great affirmation. To feel the truth of this philosophy, however, requires actually practicing the concept, noticing how every experience can be reacted to negatively or positively. It's like the "every cloud has a silver lining" saying—it may be cliché, but that doesn't mean it isn't true. Try to become grateful for the annoyances, the frustrations, the pain, the anger, the disappointment, the sadness that moves in and out of your life with as much soulful acceptance as you are grateful for the joy and love and delight you receive. It all has something to tell you. As soon as you can view a situation from a place of gratitude, all the drama and chaos melts away into acceptance. And only from a place of acceptance can you hope to find forgiveness. Gratitude is key to all things.

b. Be forgiving. Forgiveness often gets tangled up with the ego and our need to be right, or our need to seek justice, revenge, or restitution, or our need to stay miserable and victimized. Forgiveness is a very tricky thing because, like all healing, it must first begin within. If you haven't forgiven yourself, forgiving others is impossible because you cannot give to others what you do not have ourselves. You can't give love if all you have is self-hate; you can't give joy if all you have is self-loathing; you can't forgive others if you haven't forgiven yourself.

Forgiveness sometimes takes longer to find than gratitude. First of all, we often believe that forgiveness of a certain behavior validates that behavior. If these two things remain connected, forgiveness becomes impossible. When you forgive, it is not about validating the act but about letting go of the power that act has in your life. This is particularly important when it is your own act that you must forgive. We often hold ourselves accountable to a much higher standard than anyone else. This is not necessarily a bad thing, but it can become damaging when you are unable to forgive yourself for what you perceive to be your transgressions.

Thomas Moore says in his book *Care of the Soul* that soul work is messy. It doesn't happen in neat, organized little boxes. There will always be things that happen, things we do, things we say that turn out to be at best less than helpful, and at worst damaging to ourselves or others. Your job is to recognize it, redefine who you want to be, forgive yourself for being human, and move forward. It doesn't mean you condone the action but that you have the ability to tap into your own divinity, learn the lesson, and move on your path in a healthier, more enlightened, more loving manner.

When the act of forgiveness involves another party, we often believe we are doing it for the other person. Although the other party might very well benefit greatly from your act of forgiveness, it should not matter to you one way or the other. Forgiveness is about you. Until there is forgiveness, the act holds you in its grip, keeping you from moving forward. It holds your heart hostage, and thus you inadvertently perpetuate the pain of the original act. The act of forgiveness is about freeing yourself from your own grip, your own belief that you must live a miserable and damaged life because of whatever has occurred. You do not. You have the choice, in every minute you live, to move into forgiveness and free yourself to heal and become a joyous, loving, compassionate person, no matter what circumstances have occurred in your life.

Finally, you must realize that your forgiveness does not require the participation of anyone but yourself. No one else has to forgive you for your transgressions and no one has to accept your forgiveness of theirs. It is a solitary endeavor, engaged in for the sole purpose of freeing your own heart and spirit of unnecessary baggage.

So, forgive the thin-obsessed patriarchal media, knowing that their motives are all about power and money and competition and have nothing to do with you personally; and forgive yourself for taking it personally and falling prey to the manipulation. Now, reclaim your true essence and feel your heart heal from the inside out.

3. *Healing the spirit:*

a. **Stay present**: The path of gratitude and forgiveness is a much smoother one when you learn to stay more in the moment and not wander into the nether regions of the past or the unknown of the future. Nothing keeps you more grounded in non-forgiveness than holding on to the past. Learning from the past is essential. Living in the past is fatal. The NOW moment is the only one you really have. It is the only place in which you have any control. It is the only place from which you can create. Traveling any path is about one step in front of the other. If you worry about where your last step was, you will miss the step you are taking, which could mean stepping where you should not. If you look too far at the many steps you have ahead, then you will become fearful and may stop taking steps at all. Regrets of the past and fear of the future are your greatest enemies. You must be present, aware and awake in the Now in order to live your life to the fullest.

b. Release: We all have spiritual wounds; places in ourselves that have been hurt so badly or beaten down so far that they are now hidden away, fearful of coming into the sunshine. Release of grief, anger and sadness is essential in the journey toward the light. Your wounds need air and acknowledgment and awareness in order to fund the healing power you have inside yourself.

Crying is one of the quickest and most cleansing releases of grief and sadness. Give yourself permission to cry whenever you feel you need to and know that, if anyone is uncomfortable with it, it's their problem. You may not always know the reason you are needing to cry. Trust your inner self. She does a lot of work that you don't know anything about!

Another good tool for releasing anger and frustration is what I refer to as primal scream therapy, which you should try to do in a more private place. It tends to scare people! Try doing it in the car, where it can also serve as a good tool for releasing road rage! But be careful—this can hurt your throat, so don't overdo it!

Pounding pillows is still another way to release anger. Make sure you are on a soft surface, like a bed, then just let it rip, allowing the pillow to represent whatever you can identify as the catalyst of your pain.

Whatever method of release you choose, remember two things: do not direct the release at any animate object, and be gentle with yourself. You will be amazed at the relief and clarity that can come from ridding yourself of emotional toxins.

c. Play. Don't forget to play. Laugh, sing, be silly, blow bubbles, roll in the grass, run through the sprinklers or the ocean waves, play ball, have a picnic with people you love, go to a concert, have a slumber party, dance in the moonlight. Laughter is as important as crying. Remember, it's only life, after all.

4. *Search for wholeness*. It takes a great deal of courage to change how you see. It is not easy to find your true essence in this culture. And when you are not allowed to find your true self, it is very difficult to allow others to be their true selves. As always, it must begin with you. Your first step is to love every single part of who you are. Every one has something to say, something to teach you about yourself. Listen with compassion and gentleness. Some parts of you are wounded, but each has something to tell you that is very valuable to understanding your spirit and helping you see the path to joy and love. Don't endeavor to cut out those parts that are wounded, but, rather, to heal them and bring them back into the fold of your entire Being. Heal those spaces of blame, shame, guilt, fear and hate with empowerment, confidence, self-love, acceptance, and celebration.

The following visualization was designed to help women bring their body/mind/spirit together in one space. These different parts of you each have so much to give and are so much more powerful when they work together.

Find a safe, comfortable, quiet place. You may wish to tape this so you can listen more fully and attentively. If you do so, remember to speak slowly and lovingly, leaving time between each section to meditate on what comes up for you. Feel free to use some instrumental music. Relax, breathe from your belly, deep, slow breaths, letting out any tension, any expectation, any fear you might have.

WHOLENESS VISUALIZATION

We are encouraged to view our body/mind/spirit separately in this world, and now you are going to call them all into the same space with each other. Welcome them as your friends, long separated, finally reunited. Let each of them speak about where they have been, how they are now, where they want to be, how they can each help the other find their fullest self.

Start with your mind: What thoughts have been keeping you from wholeness? What beliefs do you hold about your worth in the world, your beauty, your importance? What external forces have come to bear on your perceptions of yourself? Talk to your ego/mind about changing those beliefs. Find ways to reframe those perceptions into positive affirmations, knowing that you are unique and special in this world. No one else can bring to bear the gifts you have. They are yours alone. Make up your mind to allow the world the joy of receiving your gifts and to allow you the joy of giving them.

Now, turn to your body. Has she been mistreated? Has she been starved, abused, judged, ridiculed? Have you unwittingly contributed to that? Listen to what she has to tell you. Hear her pain. Hear her desire to be loved and accepted and honored. She is your vessel. She is where you live. She is your center of power. Talk with her about how she wants to be seen; proud, strong, confident. Let her know that you will not abandon her or deny her nourishment or nurturing. Talk to her about finding ways you can love her unconditionally, no matter what anyone else says or does.

Now, turn to face your spirit. Your spirit is lovely, golden, strong, and ever patient. She is your true self. She is your pure essence. She holds all your wisdom, compassion, and love. But she requires your attention so she can help your mind find its way home to your truth, and your body feel the joy of non-judgment, acceptance and unconditional love. Ask your spirit for guidance on your journey to wholeness.

When you return from this visualization, try to find a way to express what came up for you. Create a mandala, a clay sculpture, a painting or drawing, write a poem, or simply journal.

It is impossible to separate the spiritual healing of self-love from the subjects of your body, mind, and culture. It is, in fact, the body/mind/spirit separation that requires the deepest healing. It can happen, but only as each of us heals herself. Begin with non-judgment of yourself (and then others); forgiveness of your own perceived mistakes (and then others'); shining light on your own shadows (thus allowing others to do the same); facing your fears with gratitude and anticipation (and being grateful for others who do the same); shifting your thoughts to those of abundance and joy (and thus attracting others who do the same); and knowing that you have complete power to choose your way of seeing and being.

It is in this self-knowing and taking back our power, one by one by one, that the cultural paradigm will shift and true learning and healing will begin.

Healing the Culture

From self-love flows all the goodness of the Universe
—J. Alison Hilber, 1999

Separation of life from the body is impossible. Your body is the vehicle for all that you experience. But we often find ourselves so dissatisfied with our body, that we try to dissociate from it. We may manifest this in body-size obsession, controlling our appetites for food, sex, passion, carefully monitoring our emotions, our actions, our desires. But no matter how you try, your body is still here and your dissatisfaction with it effects your mind and spirit, as well.

It is time to take back your spiritual power and move into that space of self-love and acceptance that will allow you to express your true self. Although the internal changes must come first, they cannot happen in a vacuum. In order to guard against the continuation of the cycle with each new generation, the healing of the culture is also necessary. Therefore, as you make the glorious journey toward finding your self-loving self, you must consider taking your positive, self-assured attitude boldly and visibly into the world. Turn some of your attention to the external conditions over which you may have some influence. This influence, of course, will increase in direct relation to your ability to unite with others in the effort. You remember that 11% creating the cultural shift we talked about earlier? You are it!

POWER TOOLS:

1. *Don't ignore men.* Pay close attention to the men in your life. There is a temptation in this culture to generalize and blame and speak in broad strokes when speaking of the beauty standard oppression. The oppression *is* real, the people in power *are* men. It is easy to become jaded and almost militant when raging against the system. However, women also contribute to the perpetuation of the standard and must take their share of the responsibility. Blatant generalizations not only hurt those who truly support us, but hurt us and our children, as well. It is not only female children who are culturalized in strict roles and expected behaviors. Men may seem to fare better, and, indeed, in many ways they do. But in other ways, they are just as oppressed by the patriarchy as are the women. Increase your awareness of the number of men around you who are finally "getting it." Pay attention to those men who truly support your life in positive, affirming, non-misogynist ways and reward them with praise and gratitude.

2. *Educate and encourage.* Education and encouragement are of paramount importance in any desire for change. This is most effective one-to-one. Your personal story shared with someone who is on the verge of enlightenment can be very powerful. So, share it often, and listen to their stories, as well. Understand the rules they have had to endure and lead them to the light with gentleness and compassion. There will also be plenty of those who are so stuck in the ways of their upbringing and continued culturalization that they might need a stronger hand. But remember: do not take anything personally, make no assumptions, and try not to generalize. Avoid the temptation to judge others. Everyone must come to their own truth in their own time. There may be

times when you must walk away. Feel free to do so, with your dignity and integrity in tact whenever possible.

3. *Walk the walk*. While you are elucidating the unenlightened, be sure that you are not just talking the talk. The talk is the easy part: it makes good sense and it's relatively easy to sell. But walking the walk is the hard part—that's the part that takes your courage and commitment.

For example, a few years ago I went to see a play about eating disorders. It was a great play, but all six actors were thin. The next time I saw the director, I told her that I feared that having only thin actors in the play would give a subliminal mixed message that eating disorders worked, even if they were dangerous It made me uncomfortable. She said that she agreed, but no plus-size actors had shown an interest. So, of course, when they began rehearsal again, I had to become part of the cast. I had to walk my walk, not just talk the talk. I had never acted before, but neither had many others in the cast. And we were great. There were many, many compliments about having other sizes represented and it made a big difference to many of those in the audience. So even though I was terrified of performing, I was proud to have been able to walk my walk so well.

In addition to one-on-one situations, there are myriad ways to make a statement, and very often, a difference.

♦   Stop all participation in negative body talk, whether about yourself or someone else; refrain from getting pulled into conversations that denigrate any woman's body.

♦   Do not laugh at fat jokes; and, if possible, inform the person telling the joke that it's not funny, and is, in fact, insulting.

- Complain to management when seats in public places are too small.

- Write letters to companies whose advertisements continue to perpetuate the idea that women aren't good enough just as we are (this alone should keep us all busy until the next millennium).

- Stop, stop, stop spending money on products whose main purpose is to make you feel bad about yourself; if we stop buying it, they'll stop selling it.

- Support one another and those who ally with the cause; give lots of support, lots of praise, lots of positive reinforcement.

- Most importantly, move through your life from a place of joy and confidence and self-love and abundance; remember the old saying, "living well is your best revenge." DO IT!

From Victim to Goddess

When I dare to be powerful—to use my strength in the service of my vision, it becomes less and less important whether I am afraid.

Audre Lorde (1934-1992)

You do have choices. You can continue to take in and perpetuate those pieces of the culture that tell you your body is unacceptable, or you can seek out the power of the matriarchal archetypes within us all to see the strong, beautiful, powerful woman you are. Renewing your Goddess status is easy: all it requires is remembering that you already are a goddess. But you must honor, respect and nurture those characteristics by *being* and *believing in* who it is you are and want to be.

By continuing to send us messages of scarcity and insecurity, the culture focuses our attention away from our true selves, and distracts us from the fact that we are being manipulated and controlled. None of those people telling you that you would feel better or look better or be better if you just bought this or did that or ate this cares anything about you. They are only interested in selling you something. As long as we remain in competition with each other, and with ourselves, we will continue to pour billions and billions of dollars every year into the diet, exercise and cosmetic industries. And we will continue to cooperate and perpetuate this not-so-subtle misogyny with our dollars, our energy, and sometimes our lives. It's time to stop.

Rebel against the urge to compete with other women. We need each other's support and energy and encouragement. See each other as friends and sisters, not as enemies. Give and receive validation and comfort. The word "honor" is synonymous with the concepts of respect, esteem, reverence, worship, adoration. You should certainly be feeling all of these things for yourself. And there is no reason not to feel them for all other women, as well. Our plights are so similar, no matter what our size, shape, age, ability, income, race, or sexual orientation. There is plenty of everything to go around. We live in an abundant Universe and do not need to compete with each other to get what we desire or deserve. One of the quickest ways to raise ourselves up from the place of oppression is to unite together, and turn, en masse, toward the place of power, declaring our own. In the words of African American drummer Ubaka Hill, "Women united can never be defeated."

Declare it to each other. When in the company of other women, pay attention to what they are saying. Listen with no expectations and an open heart. Encourage them to speak from their souls, and do the same yourself. Make eye contact so they know you are present and interested and available. Share your stories, be vulnerable, trust the bond that forms when you are open and willing to let the suspicions and barriers drop away. We have so much to say to each other. We have so much to learn from each other. When we begin to honor each other; when we begin to unite in our sameness and delight in our differences, knowing that we all fight the same internal and external fight; when we can look into each other's eyes, hold the gaze, and bow in reverence to the goddess energy within every one of us, then we will be able to rise above the tyranny of this culture's beauty standards.

WE ARE THE POWER IN EVERYONE

WE ARE THE DANCE OF THE MOON AND THE SUN

WE ARE THE HOPES THAT WILL NOT HIDE

WE ARE THE TURNING OF THE TIDE.

—Author unknown

The most precious gift you can give in this world is the gift of your attention, your support, and your true self. The path from victim to goddess is as simple as opening your heart and seeing yourself in others. Having experienced the empowerment of honoring and being honored, you can then turn from a place of strength and pride and confidence to the culture that works so hard to keep you down, and see it with compassion and love, thus promoting the healing process. This then becomes the energy that is manifested in the Universe and begins to multiply a thousand-fold.

You are a goddess, fueled with a fire in your belly, empowered from within, in charge of your own happiness and your own life choices. Once you decide who you are and who you want your best self to be, then every decision you make becomes an act of self-definition based on that vision. So how can you be anything but perfect?

I AM THE POWER IN EVERYONE

I AM THE DANCE OF THE MOON AND THE SUN

I AM THE HOPE THAT WILL NOT HIDE

I AM THE TURNING OF THE TIDE.

CELEBRATE YOUR BODY: Change How You See, Not How You Look

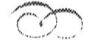

Appendix

Alison's Musings on Body/Mind/Spirit

I offer the following as nourishment for your mind, body, and spirit. Each comes forth from my own personal experience on this journey we all share toward self-love. Some of them will echo parts of the book; others will be completely new. Thank you for allowing me to share them with you.

1. Why Celebrate Your Body?

2. You Can't be a Beacon . . .

3. Will Power v. Self-Care

4. Free to Be: Thin v. Happy

5. Gratitude and Forgiveness: A Heart Healing Process

6. Emotional Poker

7. Passion is an Inside Job

8. Walk When You Want to Walk: Projections on a Snow Goose

9. Being Extraordinary

10. Walking the Path

11. Beyond Belief: Four Agreements with Your Body

Musing No. 1:

Why Celebrate Your Body?

For women, physical appearance and self-esteem are almost in-extricably connected, and most of us in this culture struggle with various body image issues, even those who actually represent society's feminine "ideal." Daily, we are battered with messages that tell us we are not thin enough, not pretty enough, not fit enough, not good enough. By internalizing these messages, we have learned to ignore our own beauty, our own worth, our own uniqueness in the Universe. Our souls are depleted and our lives become limited. Hating your body desecrates the temple you live in and is the antithesis of self-love. And self-love is the most essential element to health, joy, and spiritual growth. The goal of *Change How You See, Not How You Look Body Celebration Workshops for Women* is to help women find the inner vision and courage to ignore the rigid cultural beauty standard, and view their bodies as beautiful, powerful, sacred, and worthy of honor and respect, no matter their size, shape, or age.

A good beginning is to look at your present relationship with your body. Then you can proceed with finding a way to change the way you see, with your eyes, your heart, and your spirit. Ask yourself these questions: Are you breathing properly? Are you wearing clothes that fit? Do you pamper your body? Bathe her, lotion her, powder her, perfume her? Do you move her in ways that feel good? Stretch her? Feed her good food (including the occasional delectable things that feed your soul, as well)? Do you get her massaged? Do you have her cared for by a nurtur-ing, holistic health practitioner? Do you give her enough rest? Do you give her enough water? Do you pay attention to her flow of energy? Do you give her pleasure? Do you tell her that you love her? Do you tell her that she's beautiful? Do you believe it when others tell her she is beautiful? Do you express your grati-tude for all that she gives you and all that she does for you?

Your body is a vehicle. She needs to be given attention, be fed a properly balanced fuel, have regular check-ups, be cleaned and pampered, be protected from bumps and nicks, be well oiled to move efficiently and painlessly, and sometimes accessorized in order to show off her personality. Vehicles come in all shapes, sizes, colors, and ages. Some run smoother than others; some get a higher octane fuel; some may have been in a few more accidents or lived in a rougher neighborhood than others; some get used more than others. Where they will take you, how well they work, and how long they last depends on how well cared for they are. And that's the owner's responsibility.

Your body is like your child. She counts on you to take care of her and love her unconditionally so she can feel good about herself and show herself off with pride and self-love. She will always be there for you and will perform amazing feats at your command. However, she will not function well if abused, verbally or physically. She will become beaten down and miserable and depressed and unhappy. She may even become ill in order to get your attention. She needs you to be her protector and her champion. She needs you to shield her from outside abuse and intolerance. She needs you to give her comfort and praise. If she feels fully and unconditionally accepted by you, it will matter a lot less what anyone outside says or does. She can face the outside intolerance if she knows she is safe with you.

Your body is a temple. She deserves to be viewed and treated in a sacred manner, to be spoken to with reverence, to be worshiped as the source of your breath, your fire, your power, your life blood. Indeed, it is your body that houses your soul, and provides you a place to integrate your whole being in this physical reality so you may proceed with your life's mission.

Your body is you. She deserves to be treated with love and respect and honor, just as you do; to be celebrated for who she is right this minute, and for the space she takes up in the world. But all that must begin with you. If you don't love and celebrate her, how can anyone else be expected to? And even if they do, you won't believe them. So start right now loving your body for the precious gift she is. Stop all negative body talk. Don't ever get on a scale again. Stop spending money and energy trying to meet someone else's idea of what's "acceptable." And gather the support of other women, rather than competing against them. As African-American Drummer Ubaka Hill says, "Women united can never be defeated." You'll be amazed at the results. Changing your perspective does change your life.

© May 2000 Published in *The Onion Skin,* May 2000 (newsletter for the Onion River Coop, Burlington, Vt.)

Musing No. 2

"You Can't Be a Beacon . . . "

All together, now . . . "you can't be a beacon if your light don't shine . . . ." This little gospel song has become one of my favorite affirmations. We all have a mission in the world, but we can't pursue it well if we aren't working from a place of wholeness. Loving our bodies seems to be an especially difficult task for most women in this society. There's always something we wish was different. A lot of why that is derives from the fact that this culture encourages us to separate ourselves from our bodies. We become pieces and parts, somehow no longer connected to who we are in our hearts, our heads, and our souls. My *Body Celebration Workshops* are about finding ways to shine our light right now, without waiting to change anything. We need to remember that we are whole beings, not just our bodies. This requires changing our perceptions. There is nothing simpler and nothing more difficult.

Before we face the challenge of changing our minds and our hearts and our spirits, it helps to practice the art of living in the "now." But we need to understand that there is a difference between living *in* the now and living *for* the now. Living *for* the moment is probably the most unconscious way to live, because it demands no integrity or responsibility. Living *in* the moment requires a great deal of consciousness, awareness and focus, for the simple reason that the choices we make now have consequences. It requires choosing to forgive the past (yours and everyone else's) and release your fear of the unknown future. The future becomes known in the choices you make in the now, and in this way you have the ability to create your own reality.

Our belief systems are self-imposed, but are usually based on those which are outwardly, often indirectly, imposed upon us. Some of those beliefs about the body are: we have to be thin to be happy; we have to be beautiful to be happy; if we are fat we are lazy, stupid and have no will power; we have to be thin to be healthy; if we're fat, we're sick; if we're fat we aren't competent; if we exercise, we will always be thin; we have to be thin to exercise, etc., etc., etc. Our challenge is to release the old belief and find a new belief that lets our light shine through.

The belief we need to release is the belief that we are not perfect just the way we are. The belief we need to replace it with is that we are capable of unconditional self-love. But, because only a precious few of us are nurtured from the beginning to believe we are worthy of love at all, self-love becomes an increasingly elusive state of the soul. So, our purpose—our mission—is to courageously explore our inner beings and find that place of unconditional self-love and acceptance that will allow us to manifest love, healing, joy, abundance, and gratitude in our lives and in the world, instead of hatred, pain, misery, poverty, and anger.

One of my favorite books is called *The Key: And the Key is Willingness,* by Cheri Huber. The whole concept of "willingness" has moved me through some of the most difficult times in my life, and it is the "key" to this process, as well. We must be willing to open the door to the level of responsibility that living in the now requires, because the only way to *change* how we see is to be *responsible* for how we see. This was further illuminated for me when I recently read in *Friendship with God,* by Neale Donald Walsch, that "every act is an act of self-definition." Every choice we make in the present defines who we are and who we want to be. This kind of self-development cannot happen if we are fragmented and out of touch with the important parts of us.

And it's not about being "better." Each moment is perfect and we are perfect in it. "Growth" does not mean "better." The spiritual journey is about consciously choosing how to define our being in the world. Accepting our perfection in every moment is the key to making choices that will feed our soul and support our definition of integrity and self-love.

For me, faith is a most essential piece—faith that I will be supported in my commitment, by the Universe and by those who love me; and that I am indeed strong enough, capable enough, powerful enough, and worthy enough to make it happen. It may be slow and sometimes terrifying, but it is my faith that transforms the difficulties into challenges and the obstacles into blessings.

We are all Divine, fueled with a fire in our belly, empowered from within, in charge of our own happiness and our own life choices. Once we decide who we are and who we want our best self to be, then every decision we make becomes an act of self-definition based on that vision. So how can we be anything but perfect?

Try this visualization when you feel the need to reunite your body, mind and spirit. Close your eyes. Breathe deeply and slowly, expanding your belly with every breath. Now, ask your body if she can help you find ways to stop judging and criticizing her and begin loving her for who she is right now. Ask your mind if there are ways you are thinking that can be changed in order to view your whole being as perfect in every moment. Ask your spirit to use her patience and capacity for unconditional love to help your body and mind connect with her more often. Now visualize your body, mind and spirit all moving into the same room from wherever you have kept them. Notice how happy they are to see each other. Hear how much they have to say to each other. Feel how much more centered you are knowing that you are in a state of BEING without separation of the body/mind/spirit. Savor that feeling of joy, express your gratitude to the Universe, and let your light shine.

©July 2000 Published in *The Onion Skin,* July 2000 (newsletter of the Onion River Coop, Burlington, Vt.)

Musing No. 3

Will Power v. Self-care

During a recent Body Celebration Workshop, a woman said proudly that she had finally proved to herself that she had will power. I'm sure she expected many kudos for this accomplishment, but my first inclination was to cringe. It was another example of how twisted our self-esteem can get as a result of the media messages about the glories of "self-control" (i.e., if you don't have it, you are a slob). Her self-esteem was founded on rocky ground, however; all it would take was one moment of allowing herself the pleasure of whatever it was she was depriving herself of, and there she'd be, back in the pit of failure and self-doubt.

The concept of will power as it relates to eating is usually about dieting. Dieting is usually about deprivation. And deprivation is usually a symptom of discontent. So, already we are starting from a place of low self-esteem and unhappiness, probably built on a foundation of previous "failures." The term "will power" sets up the "good" and "bad" dualism that we humans are so fond of. We label things as good or bad so we can measure ourselves against them and thereby determine our worthiness (or more often, other people's worthiness). In this case, whether we are "healthy."

I believe that health is not determined by size, nor is it based on deprivation. In fact, the deprivation requirement is what forces the failure of most diets. We humans are strongly drawn to that which we are told we cannot have. I believe that if it wasn't drilled into us as children that sex is bad and to be avoided, most of us wouldn't have such trouble avoiding it. And then when we did decide to engage, it would be a fulfilling and wonderful experience, rather than one based on guilt and shame. The same is true with diets, which are completely based on deprivation. There are "good" and "bad" foods, and you are "good" or "bad" depending on which of them you eat. This results in guilt and shame when your natural cravings succumb to something "bad."

When you make foods good or bad, you end up making people good or bad just by what they eat. Guilt and shame are built in from the beginning of the word "diet," so how can it ever really lead you to a place of true self-love. Food is a natural comfort and necessary for survival. It is also a strong social tool, and being on a diet can severely encumber one's ability to socialize and bond with other people. You begin to bond only with others who are unhappy with themselves as well, and that cannot bring true self-love.

As usual, this culture has the cart before the horse. One cannot diet themselves to self-love. One must achieve self-love first, and then decisions about everything are made from a place of self-care, whether it's about food or sex or relationships. It no longer requires "will power." Decisions are no longer based on your ego's desire to have what it is told it cannot have. Decisions are based on a spiritual understanding of who you are and what you and your body need. Decisions are made based on choice, not on deprivation.

Will power denotes deprivation and guilt; self-care is about self-love and integrity. As long as everything you do with, put into, and say to your body is about self-care and self-love, then I say go for it. But if it's about proving you have control in your life, or proving you are capable of depriving yourself (and thus living up to that which the culture demands from you), then I say there are emotional elements at work that need to be confronted. I find that I feel better about putting healthy things in my body because I know that internally my body is working better, and I will be able to live a longer and freer life with more energy. I feel good knowing that I am capable of choosing for myself with love and nurturance, and not out of some perverse sense of obligation the culture has imposed on me. It's about finally finding my capacity for honoring my body and respecting her needs. I don't read labels for their calorie counts and serving sizes, but rather to see if they are organic or free range. I don't allow myself only certain foods at certain times of the day. The idea of waiting until dinner for the "good" stuff is all about being rewarded for your ability to deprive yourself. It also sets you up to feel like a failure if you don't follow the rules. That is not about self-care. That is about self-loathing.

All diets are about self-loathing. A *change* in your diet, i.e., deciding to eat vegetables on a more regular basis, or switching to organic yogurt, or trading in cow milk for soy milk, is different than *being on* a diet. The goal of *being on* a diet is losing a certain amount of weight in a certain amount of time, and then returning to a different way of eating. A *change* in your diet is made for the long-term and becomes part of your nutritional, self-loving self-care. I find myself craving zucchini with as much anticipation as I do chocolate. And both taste all the more marvelous for having been freely chosen.

You don't have to be on a diet to be healthy; you don't have to deprive yourself of anything in order to eat well. The concept of will power has distracted us from listening to what our bodies truly need. We must have faith in the inner wisdom which results from true self-love and naturally results in self-care.

© October 2000 Published in *The Onion Skin,* October 2000
(newsletter of the Onion River Coop, Burlington, Vt.)

Musing No. 4

FREE TO BE: Thin v. Happy

I know . . . you are used to believing that it's "thin *equals* happy." That, indeed, is what this society continues to encourage us to believe. Women especially are fed (no pun intended) great piles of misinformation, both subliminal and direct, about how being thin will change everything in our lives. Most importantly, once we are thin, we will be happy. The message being, of course, that if we are fat (or even just not what currently passes for thin), we will NOT be happy.

This strong, media-driven, patriarchal philosophy does not stop with making us unhappy with our bodies. It permeates all levels of our self-esteem. Because once we give away our power to those who would have us believe that being thin is the ultimate goal, then we have given away our power emotionally and spiritually, as well. Any time we allow others to dictate how we feel or how we see ourselves, it is because we give them the power to do so. There are not people out there who have been given the inherent ability and duty to make us feel bad about ourselves or decide who we should be and how we should look. They only have that ability because we give it to them. We, as a society, have been convinced to relinquish our own control about what's right for us to huge media groups, who then give us the answers through magazines, commercials, television, movies. Once we see what they have decided for us, we can see whether we measure up and what we must do to change so we can be just like that . . . and, therefore, happy.

As individuals, we often continue this pattern by giving this power to specific others in our lives: our family, our partner, our boss, our friends. We often even give our power to inanimate objects like mirrors, calorie counters, and numbers on a scale. We take the information we have requested from the media, and which they have so graciously and gladly provided us, and we find ways in our own world to make it true. We find people who will tell us we look bad or should really only wear dark colors or shouldn't sit in the front of the room or shouldn't say what's on our mind or shouldn't eat that double chocolate chip cookie. We scrutinize every inch of ourselves finding all the flaws; we take a perfectly fine mood and ruin it by stepping on a scale and finding ourselves lacking. We create situations whereby we begin to live limited, shameful, scared lives, afraid to be seen or heard or loved. Sure that no one out there wants to see us or hear us or love us.

This is when the media really, really has us where they want us. Because this is when they can completely sell the idea of thin equaling happy. Spiritual and emotional needs are way too fluid for the media to generalize about, but bodies are another thing. Everyone has one, everyone can perceive everyone else's. You don't have to know another thing about the person to see their body. It is the first impression, and therefore the easiest to manipulate. You can compare yourself and make all sorts of judgments without even having to say a word . . . without even making eye contact . . . without even being in the same room. Setting up standards of "beauty," whether about bodies or faces or hair or toes, is about setting up a structure by which we can all easily compare ourselves and decide whether or not we are worthy. And the more the media continues to equal thin with being worthy of love and happiness, the more we strive to go there and be that. We believe that once we achieve "thinness," we will be free from the struggle and the pain and the shame and the comparisons, and all will be well and joyful at last.

What a pile of crap! What a huge, amazingly pervasive, incredibly worshipped pile of crap! Thinness will NOT set you free. It may seemingly make you happy for a while, because suddenly all those people holding your power will be so proud that you have finally accomplished what they asked of you, that they will, for a while, shower you with adoration and praise.

So . . . now you are thin. Cool! Now what? Now you get to worry about getting fat, and what will happen to all this adoration and praise then? And will these people still love you if that happens? Oh, goddess, we can't let that happen! Wow! Sounds like more of a prison than they said being fat was!!

Now, there are many, many people out there making huge amounts of money from this media blitz about thin equaling happy. There are fitness programs, diet programs, food manufacturers, plastic surgeons, motivational speakers, authors. They are all out there using this premise of thin = happy to sell you something that will help make you thin. You just need more exercise; come spend your money with us and we'll sweat it off of you. You just need to eat less; come spend your money with us and we'll help you starve. You just need support while you exercise and eat less; come spend your money with us and we will write down the number on the scale for you every week. You just need a smaller stomach; come spend your money with us and we will completely adjust your insides so you can't hold more than 2 oz of food at a time. You just need to find out why you eat so much; come spend your money with us and we'll help you fix your emotions. Do any of these people actually care about who you are inside? Do they learn about your dreams or your hopes or your strength and courage and spiritual depth? Do they even give a damn if you are healthy? Mostly, no. They only care about making you THIN, and then providing you with more ways to spend your money to maintain that new, acceptable status. They aren't caring about whether the stress of the shame, the worry, the continuing loss of self-esteem is slowly killing your soul. As long as you look good getting there! They continue to shackle you to the idea of thin equaling happiness and therefore shackle you to their product/program/philosophy forever. Free at last??? I don't think so.

Here is what we must learn: There is no freedom in being or trying to be that which you are not. There is no freedom in trying to be a rich corporate executive if what you are is a dancer. There is no freedom in trying to be white if you are black. There is no freedom in trying to be male if you are female. There is no freedom in trying to be thin if you are not. There is only struggle and failure and depletion of your spirit. Anytime we fight against our true spirit, we will not find freedom. We can only be free by connecting with whatever Divine source we believe in, and letting it flow through us. Then we begin to feel the joy and peace and exhilaration of true freedom: the freedom with comes when we allow ourselves to be who we truly are, physically, emotionally, mentally and spiritually.

Happiness is an in-the-moment feeling that ebbs and flows with the workings of the tangible world. Joy, however, is more foundational, and is born from gratitude and self-love. Joy comes from choosing to be joyous. The contrast in the world will show you all the choices you have. And society will try to sell you what they want you to choose. But unless you give it away, only YOU have the power to decide who you are, what makes you happy in the moment, and what brings you joy inside. And those choices need to be made from your heart and soul, listening to your true source, knowing your own intrinsic value and worth in the world.

We are all born worthy and deserving of love. We do not have to earn it. We only have to choose to remember it.

©2001 Published in February 2001, in *The Onion Skin*
(the newsletter of the Onion River Coop,
Burlington, Vt.); and *Planet Vermont Quarterly.*

Musing No. 5

GRATITUDE AND FORGIVENESS:
A Heart-Healing Process

I believe that the two most powerful tools in any heart-healing process are gratitude and forgiveness. This is true whether we are healing spiritual wounds, personal wounds, or cultural wounds. My life's work is about helping heal the personal wounds caused by a thin-obsessed, patriarchal culture seemingly bent on destroying the self-esteem of its women in order to support a large portion of the economy. Specifically, my work is about guiding women on the path to self-love and acceptance of our bodies as they have been gifted to us, without the requirement of spending thousands of dollars and hundreds of hours and interminable energy on trying to look like someone else's idea of beautiful. The wounds our culture has inflicted in this regard are deep and difficult to overcome. They have left many of us living in a place of shame, guilt, blame, and self-hatred. The journey to love, acceptance and strong self-esteem requires courage, strength and faith. It also requires gratitude and forgiveness. I don't believe you can have one without the other, although they may not occur simultaneously or in any pre-ordained time frame.

It is hard to know which comes first; perhaps we must just begin with one, and the other will follow naturally. I choose to begin with gratitude, because it is a more tangible process than forgiveness. It is, for me, easier to grasp, easier to understand, easier to integrate. In Neale Donald Walsch's *Friendship with God,* he states that "gratitude is the fastest form of healing." I have this affirmation posted in my house, as I do so many others. The truth of this phrase, however, is one that must be experienced (as is the case with all things if we are to achieve full integration). It requires not only reading the affirmation, but practicing the concept. It requires that we be grateful for everything that comes into our lives. It requires that we be grateful for the annoyances, the frustrations, the pain, the anger, the disappointment, and the sadness, with as much soulful acceptance as we are grateful for the joy and love and delight we receive. As soon as we can view a situation from a place of gratitude, all the drama and chaos melts away into acceptance. And only from a place of acceptance can we hope to come to forgiveness. Gratitude is key in all things if we are to find the path to living in joy.

Forgiveness is, as I said, a less tangible concept. It, unfortunately, gets tangled up with the ego and one's need to be right, or one's need to seek justice or revenge, or even one's need to stay miserable. It also carries with it a load of dramatic religious baggage. It comes wrapped up in concepts of God and saints and holiness. When asked to practice forgiveness, people often think it is something beyond our spiritual capabilities. It is not. In fact, it is vital to our spiritual health and growth. We must free ourselves of these preconceived notions before we will be able to experience the profound freedom that comes with forgiving.

Forgiveness is a very tricky thing because, like all healing, it must first begin within. Self-forgiveness is the starting point. We cannot give to others what we do not have ourselves. We can't give love if we have self-hate, we can't give joy if we have self-loathing, we can't forgive others if we haven't forgiven ourselves.

Forgiveness often takes much longer to find than gratitude. First of all, we often believe that forgiveness of a certain behavior equals validation of that behavior. If these two things remain connected, forgiveness becomes impossible. We must be able to separate the two concepts. When we forgive, it is not about validating the act, but about letting go of the power that act has in our lives. This is particularly important when it is our own act that we must forgive. Those people who understand the necessity of taking responsibility for their choices and actions are always harder on themselves than on anyone else. We often hold ourselves accountable to a much higher standard. This is not necessarily a bad thing, but it can become damaging when we are unable to forgive ourselves for what we perceive to be our transgressions.

I don't like the concept of "mistakes," but for the purpose of this discussion, let's use it. Everyone makes mistakes. If we had the manual for life and knew all the answers, it would be pretty boring. Since we don't, we are doing the best we can with what we have, with what we know, with what we are taught. We take risks and often must go forward without all the necessary information. Thomas Moore, author of *Care of the Soul,* says that soul work is messy. It doesn't happen in neat, organized little boxes. There will always be things that happen, things we do, things we say that turn out to be, at best, less than helpful, and at worst damaging to ourselves or others. Our job then is to recognize it, redefine who we want to be, and forgive ourselves for being human. It doesn't mean we condone the action; it means we have the ability to tap into our own divinity, learn the lesson, and move forward on our path in a healthier, more enlightened, more loving manner.

When the act of forgiveness involves another party, we often believe we are doing it for the other person. Although the other party might benefit greatly from our act of forgiveness, it should not matter to us one way or the other. Forgiveness is about us. Until there is forgiveness, our hearts are held hostage, and thus we willingly perpetuate the pain of the original offending event. The act of forgiveness is about freeing ourselves from our own grip, our own belief that we must live miserable and damaged lives because of whatever has occurred. We do not. We have the choice, in every minute we live, to move into forgiveness and free ourselves to be joyous, loving, happy people, no matter what circumstances have occurred in our lives. Our forgiveness does not require the participation of anyone but ourselves. No one else has to forgive us for our transgressions, and no one has to accept our forgiveness of theirs. It is a solitary endeavor, engaged in solely for the purpose of freeing our own hearts and spirits of unnecessary burdens. It is an act of self-compassion.

The path of gratitude and forgiveness is a much smoother one when we learn to stay more in the moment and not wander into the nether regions of the past or the unknown of the future. Nothing keeps us more grounded in nonforgiveness than holding on to past behavior or events. You can't change the past, yours or anyone else's. You can, however, learn from the past. It has many, many lessons. To forget the past is to put our Now in peril, because we will be doomed to relearn the same lessons over and over. Learning from the past is essential. Living in the past is fatal. The Now moment is the only one we really have. It is the only place we have any control. It is the only place from which we can create. Regrets of the past and fear of the future are our greatest enemies. We must be present, aware and awake in the Now moment, or we are not living our lives to the fullest. Eckhart Tolle explains this concept beautifully in his book, *The Power of Now*, and I highly recommend it.

Traveling any path is about putting one step in front of the other. If we worry about where our last step was, we will miss the step we are taking, which could mean stepping where we should not. If we look too far at the many steps we have ahead, then we will become fearful, and may stop taking steps at all. Never was this concept so apparent to me as when I recently participated in a firewalk. Much of the preparation for walking the fire deals with the act of moving forward, through fear of the future, through fears the past has laden us with. One step in front of the other. The step into the fire is no different than the last step taken; it continues to move you forward. But stepping into the fire proves that we can move through the veil of limitations and boundaries we convince ourselves are impossible to overcome. Nonforgiveness is one of those unnecessary limitations we place on ourselves that keep us rooted, and make it impossible to take the step into the void. But once you make that commitment, you have no choice but to keep going forward, and suddenly you find yourself able to fly, seeing a whole new world, filled with unimaginable possibilities. This is the power of the firewalk; this is the power of forgiveness.

We all have spiritual wounds; places in ourselves that have been hurt so badly, or beaten down so far that they are now hidden away, fearful of coming into the sunshine. The wounds women have endured, and continue to endure, in the face of stringent beauty standards in this country can be healed. But it takes a great deal of awareness, diligence, and self-determination. We do have the power to change our lives; to change how we take things in; to replace self-hatred with self-love, pain with joy, feelings of loathing with the reality of knowing our own beauty. A large part of that path is forgiveness. Forgiving the patriarchy that created the standard, forgiving the men who have been taught to perpetuate and believe it, and forgiving ourselves for continuing to cooperate in helping it thrive. But wounds can only be healed in the light. They need air and acknowledgment and awareness in order to fund the healing power we all have inside ourselves. Walking the path of gratitude, forgiveness, and living in the present moment is a life-altering, life-affirming and celebratory journey. I highly recommend it.

©November 2000 Published in
Winter Issue 2000, *Planet Vermont Quarterly.*

Musing No. 6

Emotional Poker

My friend Diane said to me one day, after hearing my sad tale of returning from my childhood home with unfulfilled expectations, that the cards had all been reshuffled, and nothing was going to be in the same place now. At a time when I was profoundly confused about my emotional reactions, this analogy made a great deal of sense to me. It expressed perfectly how I was feeling: as though all my emotions, which I thought were in such a nice, neat, well-ordered pile in the middle of the table that is my life, had suddenly been picked up by a seemingly kind stranger, who said "here, let me get these ready for your next game." And before I could even begin to understand what that would mean, the deed was done. Horrified, I found that my emotions were now in no recognizable order at all. And with barely time to breathe, the next game of Emotional Poker was being laid out in front of me, with some cards face up, some cards face down, sort of like in a game of Seven Card Stud.

As I studied this phenomenon, I began to recognize the Up Cards as the emotions that are out there for the world to see; the ones that I can identify fairly quickly, either because of my own astute self-knowledge (which we have already determined is not always very reliable), or more often by my passive/aggressive behavior making itself known in the external world around me.

The Down Cards, then, are those emotions that I am aware of, but I am not ready for the world to see. They are the ones I don't really want to see, either. I peek at them occasionally, but sometimes forget that they are there; they often sit there waiting for a long time before I pay them anything more than passing attention. Then there are those that are still in the deck, waiting to be dealt. Those are the ones that are being processed at a level below consciousness . . . my soul doing her own work inside, while I am struggling with the unpredictability of the work outside. They will undoubtedly be accessible later.

My most recent escapade with the game of Emotional Poker began with the Ace of Anger and the Queen of Sadness being the top two cards tossed out on the table in front of me. How is it, I wonder, that these same cards keep getting dealt, then shuffled in for several hands, and then dealt again? Am I never finished with them? The answer, I finally admit, is No. Life, like many video games, is about moving through levels, and each hand dealt takes me deeper into my process, bringing me more contrast and, eventually, more clarity. Sometimes, cards are played swiftly, and I get to move on to the next hand with little disruption of my life. But sometimes the significance of the cards dealt overwhelms me in their attempt to penetrate whatever doors I have closed to them, and therefore they require more concentrated pondering.

During this current time of reflection, it has been difficult to contact a place of peace and centeredness. My Joy card is buried somewhere in the middle of the deck . . . I know it is there, can feel it humming softly deep inside, but it is mostly inaccessible at the moment. I know that there are several other cards to be dealt before I come upon it again. I am, for instance, expecting the Grieving card, because Anger and Sadness always lead me there. And although I know that Anger and Sadness are great teachers, I always hope that the Compassion card will also appear, because it is often followed closely by the Gentleness card, and they are both necessary on the journey from anger and sadness to grieving.

I must also remember not to put too much emphasis or energy into comparing my own hand to those of the others with whom I am playing. I can only guess at what their cards truly are. One of the cool things about Emotional Poker is that everyone can win, so competing with others is pointless and serves only as a distraction.

Now, another thing I find interesting about this game is that several different events seem to have the ability to create an instant reshuffling of the deck, even before the last hand is completed. In my case, it so happened that the last Up Card I had played before this hand was the Forgiveness card. I thought playing the Forgiveness card was the end of the game, the checkmate of life. Once I have forgiven, I thought, the pain will stop, the joy will prevail, and all will be well with my life, forever and ever, amen! Instead, I find that forgiveness is only the beginning; the front end of the journey, not the destination; it allows us to move to those deeper places with a little less fear and little more compassion, for ourselves and others. Forgiveness is the card we must draw if we have any hopes of finding the Healing card. Otherwise, we just keep pulling the Joker.

Another wonderful thing I discovered during this process is that I may not have much control over the cards I am dealt, but I do actually have access to the rest of the deck. The Shuffler is Life, and, as it turns out, She leaves the deck right there on the table so we can pull whatever cards we want from it. We may have to rummage through some uncomfortable cards to get to the ones we want, but along the way we can find the Gratitude and Faith cards, which encourage us to persevere on the search for the Joy, Bliss, Love, Acceptance cards. Or whatever other cards we each find that help us succeed with each hand that is dealt. You see, the Rules of Emotional Poker are flexible and unique to each person. And how you play your hand significantly influences the way Life plays Hers.

Here is my conclusion: I must take the cards one at a time and give them their unrushed space. I must examine each with gratitude for what they teach me, and find others that will assist and comfort me in the process. Finally, they must all get put back into the deck, with full knowledge that they will each come up again, albeit in a revised, and hopefully less scary fashion. Whether our issues are about body, mind or spirit, we usually play each new hand with a little more wisdom than the one before.

I personally find that the more open I am to the flow of life, and the more accepting I am of the inevitable reshuffling process, the more I draw those cards that support my journey. It helps to remember, too, that there is an unlimited abundance of cards in the Deck of Life, and we are all worthy of being dealt as much joy as we can handle.

©September 2001 Published October 2001 in *The Onion Skin*
(newsletter for the Onion River Coop, Burlington, Vt.).

Musing No. 7

Passion Is an Inside Job

Passion is simple and complex; focused and diverse; minute and universal; subdued and ecstatic; sacred and playful; heartful and soulful. It's something you feel and something you do. It's an emotion, an intention, a lifestyle. At least it is for me. Some people might find this to be an exhausting way to live. I think it is far more tiring to be cut off from your passionate nature, than it is to live, as I once heard someone describe it, with ferocious tenacity. Passion and intensity go hand in hand, but they shouldn't be confused with being obsessive or controlling or frantic or fearful. Passion is about feeling deeply and reverently about whatever activity you are engaged in. It is, indeed, about being fully engaged and awake. Thich Naht Hahn calls it mindfulness.

The idea of passion for me is manifest most intensely by my life's work. I remember years and years and years of feeling lost at a very core level because I didn't have a "passion" in life. Friends and family would talk about the joy of being in the garden or learning a new skill or climbing the career ladder or escaping to a quiet place to paint. Everyone seemed to have something that pulled at them, almost against their will, and joyfully consumed their energy. This was not a feeling I was familiar with, and I felt the lack of it quite poignantly. And so for all those years, I searched and longed for it. I tried to find it in my various jobs, though I always seemed to be too afraid to risk moving out of the secretarial box. I looked for it in my friendships, seeking out, sometimes desperately, those people who seemed to have already achieved this elusive goal. I took lots of classes: guitar, calligraphy, drawing. I even tried that "write children's books in your spare time" program. At last, I decided that the passion I was seeking must reside in my partner, so relationships became the sole focus of my desire, which, as we all know, is not particularly healthy for either party. It certainly wasn't healthy for me. And, bottom line: none of those things were filling that empty, nagging space.

In the early 1970s, I met someone who finally helped me see the light. She taught me that none of those yearnings were going to be met from the outside. Passion, I learned, is an inside job. Although it can be externally manifested, it begins at a soul level, that place where your true essence resides, waiting to be discovered . . . or rather, remembered. My radiant essence began to glow as I absorbed the concepts of spiritual journey, personal growth, self-knowledge, self-awareness, and unconditional love. These now are the foundation of my passionate flow. Having discovered the little trick of looking inside first, I eventually made the decision to do only that which feeds my soul, and that has led to me finding passion in nearly everything I do or feel or desire.

Interestingly, as I learned to listen to my own inner voice, I made another life-changing discovery: that passion and drama are not synonymous. Passion can be, and often is, prayerful and meditative. But for a long time, I thought that if a situation wasn't accompanied with a lot of fanfare and vocalization, it didn't qualify as possessing passion. Unfortunately, this also led to a lot more suffering and exaggeration than most situations ever deserved. The drama actually veiled the passion, and almost always led to sadness and hurt and sometimes irreparable damage. So, self-imposed drama has been nearly eliminated from my responses to the world. My little inner child occasionally misses the rush of upping the dramatic ante, and I try to listen to her rationalizations for it. But, rarely anymore does she get her own way. And she's beginning to understand that, no matter how much attention it might garner, the rush just ain't worth it anymore!

As my life philosophy grows and changes and gains clarity, one cornerstone is steadfast, and that is gratitude. Once I began the practice of living in gratitude and opening my heart equally

℘

to circumstances, whether perceived good or difficult, I also found my level of passion increase exponentially. This, to my delight, opened my senses to things to which the word "passion" had not heretofore applied in my life. Things like finally finding the perfect iron skillet for my limited cooking endeavors; stroking the soft, curly fur of my cat's belly and feeling the bubble of her purr; lingering, easy conversations with people of like mind and heart; long, more intense dialogues with people of differing perceptions; immediate connection with no need for the foreplay of small talk; appreciating the "preciousness of the unfulfilled desire" and the anticipation of its manifestation; the deep satisfaction of having a strong belief and a focused intention; those increasingly less-fleeting moments of seeing my true essence and knowing that I can do anything I choose to do; writing articles about passion, and other subjects, in hopes of touching another person's truth with my own; knowing that passion can fuel compassion and is indeed a path to unconditional love.

Finding passion in even the smallest delights has infused the intensity of finally unearthing my life's work. That which I had spent so many years envying in others began welling up inside of me during my foray back to school, and the path led me to see how everything to that point had prepared me perfectly for the manifestation of my mission. Now, I find some of my greatest joy in facilitating my body-image workshops, helping women move from the traps of hatred and shame and anger, to the havens of self-love, acceptance, and celebration.

I know that by continuing to live my life with awareness and intention, I will continue to have a passion for change, for clarity, and for the adventure of life. But I will also remember that happiness is fickle and joy is sustaining, that all things pass, and that a sense of humor is the greatest gift of all. It is only life, after all. Strive to live it passionately.

©October 2001 Published in the
Winter 2001 Issue of *Planet Vermont Quarterly.*

Musing No. 8

WALK WHEN YOU WANT TO WALK: Projections on a Snow Goose

The last Saturday in October, I decided to take a road trip to Addison, Vermont, to see the snow geese at Dead Creek Refuge. An unexplained core emotion in me is always ignited by the sound of the geese honking as they fly in often-distracted fashion over my house in Burlington's Old North End. Lounging lazily under my warm blanket, searching for motivation to get up and about, the sound of the geese approaching rockets me out of bed and (sometimes nearly naked) out to the porch, searching for and finding comfort in their consistent "V" formation and constant conversation. Is it the metaphor of migration that speaks to me, their intrinsic knowing where they must go and their unflinching and unquestioning doing of it? Is it their respect for community; their ability to communicate so deftly; their instinctual understanding that companionship and connection are key to their physical and emotional survival?

I stood in the biting wind chill, watching this glorious flock of at least 1000 birds clustered together, occasional groupings taking flight and circling overhead, sometimes finding their way back to the same spot, sometimes moving to another congregation. I stood vigil in anticipation, knowing and almost willing them to do what I most wanted to see. And within moments of my being there, they accommodated. Like an ocean of white feathers tossed into the air, the entire flock rose up, responding to some perfect, silent signal, and flew to the adjoining meadow, settling back down near the pond that was part of the wetlands. Their ascent into the air took my breath away, the reflection of the occasional bit of sunshine off their wings, the overwhelming cacophony bringing me to tears.

I looked at the meadow from which they had moved, in disbelief that every last one of them had left at the exact same moment. And as I gazed at that now empty space, I noticed, almost camouflaged, a lone goose, left standing in the middle of the pasture. From its coloring, I knew it had not yet reached maturity, so I immediately created a child's image around it. It stood perfectly still, staring intently at the spot some 100 yards away where the rest of its community had now quietly relocated. Slowly, it began to walk in their direction. As I watched it move deliberately toward its family, I continued to create the fantasy: it was a female; she was somehow injured and unable to fly; by the time she walked to the rest of the flock, they would be off for somewhere else, leaving her alone yet again; and what would happen to her when they flew permanently south, and not just in circles overhead? My heart was breaking in a million different ways. She approached a stand of tall grass leading to the wetlands area, stopped, sighed (I imagined), backed up, moved further down, turned, approached again, stopped again. My heart continued to break as I verbally encouraged her to keep moving forward, willing her across the divide. Finally, she crossed over, looking relieved, stopping to take a breath before continuing her brave journey, gazing longingly at the pond. My heart was filling up with pain at my inability to assist her, to keep her from feeling so lonely and abandoned, with my desire to whisper to her that she was not alone. She moved toward yet another stand of grass and stopped, no longer attempting to cross. And as I continued to build up this image in my mind of her being left and forgotten, I watched in disbelief as she casually flew into the air and landed softly and comfortably in the midst of the flock.

In that moment of feeling awash with relief, I realized what a perfect metaphor she was for the ways in which we project our own fears and sadness and desires onto the lives of others. Clearly, this sweet young goose had just decided to travel a little different path, for reasons that were, frankly, no one's business but her own. It was obvious that the rest of her clan was perfectly willing to allow her to do her own thing. No one came back for her or scolded her for her behavior. But I saw in her all my own childhood feelings of loneliness, abandonment, and not fitting in.

But my childhood abandonment issues were not the lesson. I have long ago acknowledged them and continue my reparenting each and every day. The lesson was that judging another person's experience and making assumptions from a distance is a very dangerous and unloving thing to do. It further deepened my understanding that each person must be allowed to live her or his life from their own true essence, and that everyone else's view of that life is veiled with their own projections and perceptions and life experiences. I stood there in the road, laughing at myself for having so thoroughly wrapped this bird's experience up in my own soulful issues. She just wanted to take a little walk, most likely a meditation that I perceived as sadness. Now I am able to view it as an act of courage, not despair; self-knowledge, not loneliness; self-love, not fear.

All of us have our own path to walk. Sometimes it will fit relatively well into the formation of those around us; sometimes it will divert drastically from the crowd. Whatever we decide to do, whatever road we decide to follow, as long as we are guided by our true essence, we are always on the right path. And no one else's projection, no matter how well-intentioned, can pierce our "knowing" of our truth. As I walked a labyrinth later in the day, feeling immense gratitude for my magical experience, I felt this mantra well up: Walk when you want to walk, fly when you want to fly. Stay centered on your own path, and have compassion for the well-meaning spectators.

©October 2001 Published in the
Winter 2001 Issue of *Planet Vermont Quarterly*.

Musing No. 9

Being Extraordinary

In celebration of my fiftieth birthday . . . or as Thich Naht Hahn calls it, my fiftieth Continuation Day . . . I hosted a firewalk. Yes, I mean an event where you actually walk across coals burning at 1200° or more, protected only by a strong belief and a focused intention. Twenty of my friends accepted the invitation, some with cynicism, some with excitement, some with fear, all with curiosity. The whole foundation of walking on fire, at least as presented by Heather Rice (a firewalker and human being beyond compare), is not to learn how to walk on fire, but to learn how to walk through fear and move beyond the beliefs that limit us, especially the belief that ordinary people cannot do extraordinary things. So the fear portion of everyone's reaction was actually the perfect emotional space to be occupying. Less than half of those accepting the gift of this opportunity expressed any interest in actually touching toe to glowing coal. But still they came . . . they even paid money.

The vessel for our magnificent journey was the grounds of a magnificently sacred space in Monkton, Vermont. It was a gloriously beautiful day, sparkling blue sky, warm breeze, bright sun. I unabashedly took full credit for this day dawning in such glory, since I know it manifested out of the 14 months of pure intention that had gone into the creation of this event. Arriving just before sunset, we were treated to a horizon of thickening clouds, parting to allow the sun to crash through in bold and striking beams of golden light across the purple mountains. As a very special Catholic friend of mine said many years ago of one of the many sunsets we shared together, it looked just like a holy card. It was Holy, indeed. Against this wondrous sky, some people walked the incredible stone labyrinth, one of two created in the name of the goddess. One by one, two by two, my friends descended upon this sacred land, gathering together for the first time . . . many having never known each other except through my storytelling. As I greeted each of them, I could feel the energy intensify, within and around me.

For the better part of the evening, we were ensconced in a twelve-sided adobe-like building, with several tiny windows whose ledges held stones, flowers, and other offerings from the Earth. Heather began, drawing each of us in with her passion, her playfulness, her joy in what she does. And drawing each of us out—out of ourselves, out of our wariness, out of our skepticism, into a world of possibility, opportunity, and choice. We were treated to stories and exercises that mesmerized us, made us laugh, opened our souls, and brought us face to face with our own potential.

As I sat and listened to the presentation, I was extremely mindful that the room was filled with people I love, people with whom I am connected at various depths, for various reasons, for various lengths of time. One woman I have known less than two years; two others have been in my heart since I was 20. All of them share my life, each as important as the next, each as loved as the other. And by the end of the evening, their fear, cynicism, doubt and curiosity were transformed into self-empowerment. I believe that each person left having rediscovered a part of themselves they had not known before . . . a beautiful, strong, courageous, magnificent self; the self that drew me into their lives in the first place, and keeps me ever present for them.

The true miracle of that night for me, however, was not that by the end of the evening almost every person joyously danced on the fire, or that even those who didn't made a powerful choice that honored their true selves in that moment. It was not the glorious sunset, the Divine synchronicity, the precious experience of a long held desire manifested beyond my vision, or even the reiteration of the absolute wonder and support of the Universe in all that I do. The miracle . . . the extraordinariness of that evening, and that which I will remember even into my next 100 lifetimes . . . is the love.

As person after cherished person rose to express their intentions for being present, each came forth with words of honor, respect and love for who I am and have been in their life. One after another showered me with pearls of their own true essence, confirming and honoring the connection of our lives. And the most precious gift I gave myself that night was the gift of surrender—surrender to my own worthiness; to my own perfection; to my own power to touch other people's hearts and souls and willingness to allow mine to be touched in return. The miracle was finally understanding that the greatest proof that one has achieved unconditional self-love is when one can surrender to the love of others, taking it in with pure and undiluted joy and the knowledge of the truths it expresses.

So, for all the extraordinary things that occurred that night, it is the love I will always hold in my core: the love I felt witnessing each person admit their fear and then boldly walk through the veil, recognizing, maybe for the first time, their own power, their own potential, their own truth. It is my fondest hope that they also felt and surrendered to the love that I returned to them that night, and indeed return to them in every moment of every day.

Buddhists speak of non-attachment. I have always struggled with the meaning of this philosophy, even as I embrace so many of the Eastern teachings. I discovered that night that there is nothing in life as uplifting as the sharing of unconditional love. And it is the "unconditional" part, I believe, that embodies the nonattachment concept. Love without condition, without judgment, without boundary, for everyone around you and most specifically for yourself. This is what allows us to move boldly through life, taking each next step through whatever challenge is presented, knowing we can do anything we choose.

Someone said to me, "well, that's an experience it will be hard to beat." But that would mean that the best is behind me. And I know that to be false. For, the truth I hold in every memory of every startling moment of that night is that I live in a state of grace, each expression and celebration of which buoys all future experiences to their highest potential. The best is not behind me, and the best is not to come. The best is right now.

©November 2001

Musing No. 10:

Walking the Path

Despite the plentitude of machine gun fire and exploding glass buildings, "The Matrix" is a movie that also has a strong and well-defined spiritual theme. Basically, it's about being faced with obstacles that force you to define who you believe yourself to be and then funding the strength and courage to BE it. It is a line from this movie that inspired the title of this article: "Knowing the path is different from walking the path." It is no coincidence (as nothing is) that I recently watched bits and pieces of this movie every time it appeared on television over the course of a month. Why I was so drawn to seeing it over and over was a puzzle to me, but it didn't stop me from seeking it out whenever I saw it in the TV guide. It wasn't long before I was offered some clarity on the matter. Bear with me.

On the Thursday evening before Solstice, I attended a women's restorative yoga celebration during which we ac-knowledged the goodness of the light *and* the dark and the perfection and necessity of both in our lives. In closing the circle, we shared a blessing, to which we were invited to add our own thoughts: "may I be happy, may I be peaceful, may I be free." I added "may I be loving." I hadn't thought about it, it just was what I wished, not only for myself but for everyone else. It seemed that to be more loving would facilitate the happiness, peace and freedom. It was a powerful meditation for me.

In the book *Friendship with God*, Neale Donald Walsch contends that whenever we define how we wish to be in the world, we are immediately presented with contrast to help clarify the truth of our desire. So it should have come as no shock to me that the day following the Solstice celebration, an event occurred which resulted in a rather venomous, unprovoked verbal attack on me. The tirade shocked me and, although the person created the conflict, she refused the confrontation, so I was in the dark about what wrong she thought I had perpetrated. Besides dismay and confusion, my immediate response was anger, provoked not just by this incident, but by the pattern of behavior it represented. I said nothing to her, for, besides there being no opportunity, I also knew it would be useless considering the level of anger on both sides. I did, instead, seethe, not just in the moment, but for most of the four days of the holiday. I found myself in constant self-dialogue, conjuring up all of the equally venomous things with which I could retaliate in self-defense. Always within this dialogue, however, was another voice saying "why are you letting this person disrupt the peace of your life? Why are you taking this in so deeply when you know that it is about her and not you?"

After two days of relentless bickering in my head, the truth finally dawned: I was taking it so seriously because it *WAS* about me. She had definitely created the conflict, but my *reactions* to her were completely mine to own. She was, indeed, the Universe's expression of contrast in my life. Had I not just the night before contended that I wished to be more loving in the world? Did it not make perfect sense, then, that I would be faced immediately with a situation that one could easily convince themselves deserved retaliation? Another tenet of *Friendship with God* is "every act is an act of self-definition." Having taken this edict to heart in recent months, I was faced with this choice: to respond from my ego, with full justification, or to respond from loving compassion, with no justification except that it is who I choose to be. Which response did I want to define me?

I rarely struggle anymore with knowing what I believe or how I want to be. My challenge comes in remaining centered and self-loving enough to actually BE that which I believe and want. It has become crystal clear to me that, whereby my first 50 years were about learning my path, my next 50 years are slated to be about walking my path. However, most of us know that it's not an easy transition to make. The ego can be extraordinarily seductive when one is attacked, especially when it is seemingly undeserved. But the ego is only interested in being right; the soul is interested in being happy. The majority of people choose to sacrifice happiness for being right because being right feels really good for a few minutes. But when being right results in the continuation of a tense, spiteful, hateful, contentious situation, then what good can come from it? Besides, perception is reality, so my idea of right isn't necessarily anyone else's. I profess to believe in leading from the soul, not the ego, so what was I going to do here? Was I going to follow the easy path of returning venom with venom, a path I knew I was fully capable of walking, or was I going to look deep inside myself and find the compassion necessary to understand the fear and misery from which the attack was born and a way to respond from a loving space? After all, I thought, if I talk about my path but am unable to do the actual work, then all I am is a chatter box with nothing real to offer myself or others.

It's so very easy to be loving to those I love and who love me back. However, I know that being loving toward those who are irritating, annoying, contrary, angry, hateful or bitter is a much more difficult task, especially if it's aimed at me. I am much more likely to be lured into a place of defensiveness and retaliation, which only furthers the conflict and rarely allows for figuring out the true motives involved. I do believe in justice, but justice can be achieved without vengeance. I can establish boundaries and hold people responsible for their actions without making them bad people and without taking any of it personally. This does not mean I have to invite them into my fold of intimate connections. It merely requires that I try to hold them in a vessel of compassion and understanding for whatever pain and fear causes them to be in the space they are.

Journeying through this event also solidified another of my philosophies which must be walked as well as talked . . . living in gratitude. That means being grateful for everything, no matter how unfair or unwarranted or tragic or painful it may be. Rather than making myself the victim of this woman's acting out, it was more productive and loving to accept it with gratitude for what it taught me about myself and the choices it forced me to clarify. Once I realized that I was obsessing over the incident not because it was so unfair, but because the Universe had presented it as a necessary tool on my path of continued self-knowledge, I laughed and cried. It was a relief and a joyous revelation!

Understanding the difference between knowing the path and walking the path is a daily practice that is important both personally and professionally. Those of us who choose to help others on their journeys must be especially vigilant about doing our own work. We must take responsibility for our own path before we can proffer any assistance to others. Clarity about our own motives, defenses and ego is essential to reducing the amount of projection we give off and take in. We teach what we most need to learn and the best way to teach is by example. The more time I spend facilitating my workshops, the more time I must spend doing the same work myself. In all circumstances of my life, it is no longer enough just to know the path; I must always endeavor to walk the path.

©January 2002

Musing No. 11

BEYOND BELIEF: Four Agreements with Your Body

One of the most impactful concepts in my life over the past few years has been "don't take anything personally." This philosophy comes from one of my favorite books, *The Four Agreements,* by don Miguel Ruiz. The basic tenet of the book is that, from birth and sometimes before, we are taught our beliefs by others, and by living according to those beliefs, we have tacitly agreed to their truth. Ruiz believes there are only four agreements necessary to live a joyous, integrous and spiritually fulfilling life. They are:

(1) Be impeccable with your word.

(2) Don't take anything personally.

(3) Don't make assumptions.

(4) Always do your best.

These four agreements have proven invaluable to me, not only in navigating through the external world, but in training my mind to think differently about myself. Since the foundation of my work in the world involves helping women create a strong, loving body image, I began ruminating on how these four agreements could specifically relate to the journey toward self-acceptance and love.

(1) *Being impeccable with your word* is about speaking from your truth at all times and that you don't speak from a mean, spiteful, blaming or hateful place. That means there can be no more negative body talk or badmouthing about your Body or yourself. It has always amazed me how much more critical we are of ourselves than of anyone else. There are things you would never say to another person, but have no problem rattling off in your own self-dialogues without a second thought. Things like,

"you're so ugly," or "you're so fat," or "you shouldn't even leave the house looking like this," or "you're so stupid."

That kind of negative energy and spiteful self-talk is very damaging. Because your mind/body/spirit are inseparable parts of your true essence, you cannot berate one without it affecting the others. Continuing to hate yourself in any way will lead to an unhappy mind, an ailing body, and a wounded spirit. On the other hand, walking the path toward self-love will create equally buoyant results on all levels. You will find yourself feeling free, healthy and joyful. As you choose to be impeccable with your word toward yourself in these very tangible ways, you will find it much easier to be the same with others in your life, as well.

(2) *Not taking anything personally* is knowing that when other people say things about you that are hurtful or judgmental, whatever they say is not about you, it is about them and comes from their own fears and past experiences. There is no "capital T" Truth to be had, because everything is seen through our own personal perception of reality. What offends one person, won't offend another. What feels good to one person may feel bad to another. Understanding this concept of "perception is reality" is very helpful in moving out of the belief that everyone else's world revolves around us, and that everything they do and say is a personal affront—or personal compliment—to us. People's reactions to who we are, what we do, or how we look have little or nothing to do with our truth of who we are, what we do, or how we look. It has only to do with what judgments that person's experience and beliefs have formed. Bottom line: it's not about you, it's about them.

Someone who tells you you need to change the way you look or behave is either jealous, fearful, uneducated, or trying to make a buck off your dissatisfaction. The media wants you to be unhappy so you will spend your money trying to find happiness. People want you to be like them because it's often the only way they have to judge who they are. When their beliefs are challenged, people will make whatever judgment is necessary to support their cherished belief systems. For instance, if you are fat and happy, people will make judgments that you are in denial, because their belief is that you can't be fat and happy at the same time. That judgment has nothing to do with you and everything to do with them. So, don't take anything personally. Even the good stuff isn't really about you, but about what makes them feel better. Good for you! Take it in and enjoy it. But don't let it go to your head.

The other side of this agreement is that you also realize that your reactions to other people are about you, not about them. You reacting ashamed and ugly because someone tells you you are ugly or fat or stupid is because somewhere inside of you, you have a belief that they are right. If your reaction is to shrug it off and ignore their judgment, it's because inside yourself you have a belief that they are wrong. Whatever reaction you have, it's about you and cannot be blamed on or credited to anyone else.

Life gets extraordinarily better once you don't take anything personally and are responsible for your own reactions without blaming or becoming a victim. It has brought about an amazing transformation in my world view that has benefited me "beyond belief," because it changed my belief.

(3) *Making no assumptions* is perfect for helping you open up to those people who show you attention and say they love you. So often our own self-hatred closes us off to those who do love us because we assume that they couldn't possibly be telling us the truth. This is where our own beliefs become self-fulfilling prophecies. Never assume anything based on your past experience. You can be cautious, if you must, but always leave the door open to the possibility of something magical and serendipitous. Not everyone in this patriarchal society buys into the culture's obsession with thinness or the idea that physical appearance reigns above all. In fact, I believe that the media leads us to believe this is far more true than it is. Therefore, let go of any assumptions you have about not being good enough and allow

yourself to experience the love, affection, and attention that is all around you.

(4) *Always do your best.* The important thing about this agreement is that it encompasses not only trying your best, but then moving on without regret or second guessing your decisions. If you try your best and look back without regret, you eliminate the temptation to punish yourself for your perceived failures. Many women try to look like super models and most women fail, because it is not who they are. This, however, is not a failure. It is simply a lesson in self-acceptance. Trying to be the best person you are, living your own truth, in your own uniqueness of body, mind and spirit, is the most important agreement you can make with yourself. Then, there are no failures and no regrets and no punishments.

It is very important to remember as you travel the path to self-love and acceptance that there may be moments of frustration when it feels like you aren't making any progress or are backsliding. These moments are perfect lessons in self-forgiveness, and therefore can't be characterized as backslides because they actually serve to move you forward. They are perfect practice for nonjudgmental, unconditional love and acceptance of yourself in every moment.

I urge you to begin considering how these agreements might impact all phases of your life, starting with your relationship with your Body. She deserves to be spoken to and about with reverence and love. She deserves to know that what other people say about Her is about them and shouldn't be believed. She deserves to have the opportunity to be loved without assumptions that She is not lovable getting in the way. She deserves your trying your very best to love, accept and protect her, and never regret who She is. She deserves to be loved "beyond belief."

©February 2002

References

American Heritage Dictionary, 3d ed., 1994.

Barnett, Lynn and Chambers, Maggie. *Reiki Energy Medicine: Bringing Healing Touch into Home, Hospital, and Hospice.* Rochester, Vt.: Healing Arts Press, 1996.

Bardo, Susan. *Unbearable Weight: Feminism, Western Culture, and the Body.* Los Angeles: Univ. Of Calif. Press, 1993.

Bernell, Bonnie. *Bountiful Women. Large Women's Secrets for Living the Life They Desire.* Berkeley: Wild Canyon Press, 2000.

Blank, Hanne. *Big Big Love: A Sourcebook on Sex for People of Size and Those Who Love Them.* Emeryville, Calif.: Greenery Press, 2000.

Blank, Hanne. *Zaftig: Well Rounded Erotica.* San Francisco: Cleis Press, 2001.

Brannon-Quan, Tami and Licovoli, Lisa. *Love Your Body. A Guide to Transforming Body Image.* Newport Beach, Calif.: Esteem Publishing, 1996.

Brown, Laura & Rothblum, Esther. *Overcoming Fear of Fat.* New York: Harrington Park Press, 1989.

Chodron, Pema. *The Wisdom of No Escape and the Path of Loving Kindness.* Boston: Shambhala, 1991.

Chodron, Pema. *When Things Fall Apart.* Boston: Shambhala, 1996.

Cooke, Kaz. *Real Gorgeous.* New York: W. W. Norton & Co., 1996.

Erdman, Cheri. *Nothing to Lose: A Guide to Sane Living in a Large Body.* San Francisco: HarperCollins, 1995.

Erdman, Cheri. *Living Large.* San Francisco: HarperCollins, 1996.

Gilman, Susan Jane. *Kiss My Tiara: How to Rule the World as a Smartmouth Goddess.* New York: Warner Books, 2001.

Hendricks, Gay and Kathlyn. *Conscious Loving: The Journey to Co-Commitment.* New York: Bantam Books, 1990.

Higgs, Liz Curtis. *"One Size Fits All" and Other Fables.* Nashville: Thomas Nelson Publishers, 1993.

Hill, Ubaka. *Shapeshifters* (audio CD), 1995.

Hirschmann, Jane and Munter, Carol. *When Women Stop Hating Their Bodies: Freeing Yourself from Food and Weight Obsession.* New York: Fawcett Columbine, 1995.

Huber, Cheri. *The Key. And the Name of the Key is Willingness.* Mountain View, Calif.: A Center for the Practice of Zen Buddhist Meditation, 1984.

Jonas, Steven and Konner, Linda. *Just the Weigh You Are: How to be Fit and Healthy Whatever Your Size.* Shelburne, Vt.: Chapters, 1997.

Manheim, Camryn. *Wake Up! I'm Fat!* New York: Broadway Books, 1999.

"The Matrix" (film). Barrie Osborne (Ex. Producer), Warner Bros., 1999.

Moore, Thomas. *Care of the Soul.* New York: HarperCollins, 1994.

Newman, Leslea. *SomeBody to Love: A Guide to Loving the Body You Have.* Chicago: Third Side Press, 1991.

Northrup, Christiane. *Women's Bodies, Women's Wisdom.* New York: Bantam, 1994.

Northrup, Christiane. *The Wisdom of Menopause: Creating Physical and Emotional Health and Healing During the Change.* New York: Bantam, 2001.

Pipher, Mary. *Reviving Ophelia. Saving the Selves of Adolescent Girls.* New York: Ballantine Books, 1994.

Reilly, Patricia Lynn. *Imagine a Woman in Love with Herself.* Berkeley: Conary Press, 1999.

Richardson, Brenda Lane and Rehr, Elane. *101 Ways to Help Your Daughter Love Her Body.* New York: Quill, 2001.

Ruiz, don Miguel. *The Four Agreements.* San Rafael: Amber-Allen Publishing, 1997.

Ruiz, don Miguel. *The Mastery of Love.* San Rafael: Amber-Allen Publishing, 1999.

Hicks, Esther and Jerry. *Science of Deliberate Creation* (audio programs). Houston: Abraham-Hicks Pub., 2000.

Sherman, Rita. *How to be Yourself.* New York: HarperCollins, 1992.

Stuart, Mary S. and Orr, Lynnzy. *Otherwise Perfect: People and Their Problems with Weight.* Deerfield Beach, Fla.: Health Communications, Inc., 1987.

Tolle, Eckhart. *The Power of Now. A Guide to Spiritual Enlightenment.* Novato, Calif.: New World Library, 1999.

Walsch, Neale Donald. *Friendship With God.* New York: G.P. Putnam's Sons, 1999.

Wann, Marilyn. *FAT!SO?* Berkeley: Ten Speed Press, 1998.

Webster's Collegiate Thesaurus. Maire Weir Kay, ed. Merriam Webster, Inc., 1988.

Weil, Andrew. *Breathing: The Master Key to Self-Healing* (audio cassette). Louisville: Sounds True, 1999.

Weil, Andrew. *Eating Well for Optimum Health: The Essential Guide to Food, Diet & Nutrition.* New York: Knopf, 2000.

Weiner, Jennifer. *Good in Bed: A Novel.* New York: Pocket Books, 2001.

Wiley, Carol. (ed). *Journeys to Self-Acceptance: Fat Women Speak.* Santa Cruz: The Crossing Press, 1994.

Williamson, Marianne. *A Return to Love: Reflections on the Principles of A Course in Miracles.* New York: HarperCollins, 1992.

Williamson, Marianne. *A Woman's Worth.* New York: Ballentine Books, 1993.

Wolf, Naomi. *The Beauty Myth: How Images of Beauty are Used Against Women.* New York: William-Morrow, 1991.

About the author

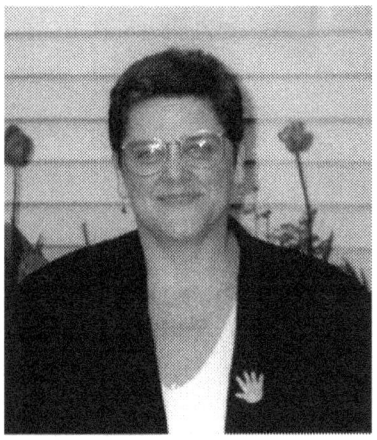

J. Alison Hilber has a B.A. in Transpersonal Psychology from Burlington College, and is dedicated to helping women on the path to joyous celebration of their bodies through her *Change How You See, Not How You Look Body Celebration Workshops for Women* and this book. Alison lives in Burlington, Vermont, with her cat, Psyche, who is a daily reminder of the delights of having a soft, round belly.

To contact Alison or for further information about the workshops:

J. Alison Hilber
P.O. Box 1841
Burlington, VT 05402

alison@changehowyousee.com
www.changehowyousee.com

www.ingramcontent.com/pod-product-compliance
Lightning Source LLC
Chambersburg PA
CBHW020527290526
45786CB00002B/783